DATE DUE

DEC 0 1 1995	
NOV 2 5 2000	
NOV – 6 2003	
GAYLORD	PRINTED IN U.S.A.

HEALTH IN THE MEXICAN-AMERICAN CULTURE

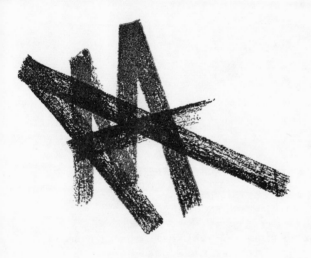

HEALTH IN THE MEXICAN-AMERICAN CULTURE

A Community Study
by Margaret Clark
University of California Press
Berkeley, Los Angeles, London

UNIVERSITY OF CALIFORNIA PRESS
BERKELEY AND LOS ANGELES, CALIFORNIA
UNIVERSITY OF CALIFORNIA PRESS, LTD.
LONDON, ENGLAND

SECOND EDITION
SECOND PRINTING, 1973
ISBN: 0-520-01668-8
PRINTED IN THE UNITED STATES OF AMERICA

For my parents MYRTICE *and* C. A. CLARK

PREFACE TO SECOND EDITION

In the ten years since this study was first published many changes have occurred both within Mexican-American communities and between ethnic minorities and American society at large. The barrio of Sal si Puedes no longer exists as it did during the 1950's; most of the houses have been razed in the wake of an urban renewal program. The people of the barrio, however, are still living in California

A few families have realized their hopes of a less precarious life, a little further away from the grip of poverty—a better house, a steady job, and an opportunity to keep their children in school a few years longer. Many others, however, have simply pushed out into other barrios not unlike the old, or have joined the ranks of the urban poor in the ghettoes of California cities. If they are like Spanish-speaking families in other parts of California, many still struggle with the same problems they faced ten years ago—uncertain employment, low income, substandard housing, and inadequate medical care.

The number of Mexican-American families in California has increased greatly within the past decade. A part of this growth is simply a reflection of general population increase, but another part is the result of continued in-migration from Mexico, especially to the southern part of the state. The new migrants, most of whom entered the country in the fifties and early sixties, have reinforced the Latin-American character of California barrios—a whole new generation of Spanish-speaking children are facing the problem of trying to acquire an education in Anglo-American schools.

The past decade has also seen a major change in the relationships between the Spanish-speaking community and Anglo-American society. The social and political ferment of recent years has broken down some of the old isolation that formerly characterized California barrios. Community leaders, social action groups, and student organizations have emerged as ever stronger forces demanding attention to the social and economic evils that have beset the poor for generations. Health and medical agencies have responded to some degree by adding Spanish-speaking professionals to their staffs and by attempting to establish new modalities of health care. Much more needs to be done, however. Mexican-American communities still do not have adequate medical facilities. Clinics are overcrowded and understaffed; most families do not have health insurance and can be bankrupted by soaring costs of hospital services and doctors' fees; crippling disabilities go untended; many children are inadequately fed and clothed; psychiatric care, except for the most seriously disturbed, is still largely unavailable to the poor; there are still far too few Spanish-speaking doctors, nurses, and other health professionals.

Although the study reported in this book was conducted years ago, many of the problems it raises still prevail. For this reason I hope it will continue to be of some use to people working in medical and public health programs.

There is a second reason, too, that I again offer this work to readers. The ethnic culture describe here is disappearing to some extent in California; at least it is rapidly changing. Yet, this is the background from which many of today's Californians of Mexican descent have come. I hope, if any of them read it, that they will see more than a collection of quaint folkways. I hope they will recognize and respect a way of life rich in history, filled with unsung heroism, and based on lasting values of caring and sharing; that they will recoognize the enormous energy and ingenuity of their parents and grandparents—proud and durable people too often beleaguered or ignored by an alien majority. *La raza*— the people of Sal si Puedes—will endure.

To AN EXTENT *unknown in history, people today are being asked, or given the opportunity, to accept new ideas and practices, attitudes and habits. Often, acceptance of the new means that the old must be given up; the two may be mutually incompatible. People are influenced in their decision to accept or reject the new, to abandon or cling to the old, by their cultural background, which gives them a value system justifying their likes and dislikes, beliefs and attitudes, customs and habits. From their cultural background likewise comes an understanding of their own proper behavior and of the behavior which they may logically expect from others in social situations.*

Personnel of programs which have as their goal significant improvements in health, education, and social welfare, among people of ethnic origins distinct from their own, increasingly find that information on the cultural backgrounds of these people facilitates their work. For improvements imply that old, and often cherished, beliefs and ways may have to be given up for new ones.

The study on which this book is based was designed to secure sociocultural information that would be helpful to professional persons in the United States working with people of Mexican background who have not yet been fully assimilated into American Culture. Although the study focused particularly on public health problems, data were gathered and conclusions drawn that are applicable to related fields, such as curative medicine, education, and social welfare.

The field research for this book was made possible by a grant from the Rosenberg Foundation of San Francisco. The Foundation also underwrote part of the cost of publication. The following committee of public health and social science specialists planned and supervised the work and dispersed the grant: Ralph L. Beals, Professor of Anthropology and Sociology, University of California, Los Angeles; George M. Foster, Professor of Anthropology, University of California, Berkeley (Committee Cochairman and Field Director); Mrs. Ann Wilson Haynes, Chief, Bureau of Health Education, California State Department of Public Health (Committee Cochairman);

David G. Mandelbaum, Professor of Anthropology, University of California, Berkeley; Dorothy B. Nyswander, Professor Emeritus of Public Health, University of California, Berkeley; W. Elwyn Turner, M.D., Director, Santa Clara County Health Department, San Jose, California.

Mrs. Leslie M. Ganyard, Executive Director of the Rosenberg Foundation, was a helpful participant in Committee meetings. Selected members of the staff of the Santa Clara County Health Department met with the Committee and contributed significantly to the project by indicating areas for inquiry in which they recognized practical problems.

The Committee decided that the problems of health and culture on which it hoped the research would shed light could best be studied in the Spanish-speaking enclave called Sal si Puedes, an unincorporated community on the eastern edge of San Jose, in Santa Clara County, California. Miss Clark, then a graduate student in anthropology at the University of California, Berkeley, was employed in November, 1954, to make the basic study. Dr. Thomas McCorkle, an anthropologist, was employed in June, 1955. In addition to gathering the data, Dr. McCorkle served as Field Director for ten weeks during Professor Foster's absence. Both Dr. Clark and Dr. McCorkle remained in the field until the end of 1955.

During the first phase of the study, a general sociocultural analysis of the community was made. Information, obtained by standard ethnographic techniques, included a census, the use of open-ended interviews of persons with representative characteristics of the group, informal but intensive observations of family and community life, and direct participation in many social and religious activities. Approximately 65 per cent of the families of Sal si Puedes were surveyed in the ethnographic census, and approximately 20 per cent were interviewed intensively in this part of the study. Public health problems received primary attention in the second phase of the field research. Traditional systems of folk medicine, ideas of disease causation, home remedies, and the role of folk medical practitioners were studied. Relations between public health personnel and Spanish-speaking people were observed in homes and clinics, and Mexican-American patients were interviewed in hospitals and sanatoriums, in order to obtain information on how clients feel about medical, hospital, and public health service.

This book is based on Miss Clark's doctoral dissertation (Sickness and Health in Sal si Puedes: Mexican-Americans in a California Community). Dr. McCorkle's field data were drawn upon for both the dissertation and this book. The Committee acknowledges with pleasure his significant contribution to the project.

CONTENTS

149-61

xiii

HEALTH, the prevention of illness, and the curing of disease constitute a major area of interest to the peoples of all cultures. No human group lacks an explanation of the conditions that must be fulfilled or maintained for the individual to enjoy good health, and no human group lacks explanations of the causes of illness. No human group is so simple but that it has social, religious, and clinical devices to cope with illness—ceremonies to frighten away demons, magical rites to recover a lost soul, herbal remedies to cure a variety of ailments, and physical and surgical manipulations to repair broken bones and other injuries.

No medical system (that is, a complex of ideas about causes and cures of disease) is entirely rational, and none is entirely irrational. Any medical system, whether based on the scientific knowledge and practices of modern medicine or on the superstitions and empirical knowledge of primitive groups, is at least a reasonably coherent and unified body of belief and practice. Since curing practices are a function of the beliefs on the nature of health and the causes of illness, most curative procedures are understandable and "logical" in the light of those beliefs.

Medical beliefs in all cultures are among those held to most tenaciously. Many of these beliefs become firmly engrained in the minds of people during childhood, and the emotional quality attached to them is almost sacred. Moreover, the stress of illness and the ever-present fear of death are not conducive to "rational" action, if by "rationality" one means the abandonment of old and tried and true procedures for new and little-understood treatments.

Since medical systems are integral parts of the cultures in which they occur, they cannot be understood simply in terms of curing practices, medical practitioners, hospital services, and the like. Medical systems are affected by most major categories of culture: economics, religion, social relationships, education, family structure, language. Only a partial understanding of a medical system can be gained unless other parts of culture can be studied and related to it.

Whenever individuals from one culture, with their particular beliefs about health, illness, and the prevention and cure of disease, come to live as members of a minority group within another culture which has a vastly different medical system, emotional and social conflicts often result when illness brings members of the two groups together. Conflicts resulting from culture contact are not, of course, confined to medical relations. Similar conflicts arise in other areas of life when people, in contact with a culture other than their own, find it necessary to make significant changes in many of their ways of living and thinking. Medical changes are merely one phase of the larger process of acculturation.

Sometimes, however, medical conflicts are particularly disturbing, and their resolution may require special attention. Immigrant peoples in the United States often find themselves without the full spectrum of medical resources they had in their native lands. They may have no access to traditional ways of dealing with illness, and the healing methods commonly practiced in the United States may seem strange and frightening. Yet if members of ethnic minorities do not follow the health rules imposed on other residents (compulsory vaccination, isolation of contagious diseases, environmental sanitation), they may become a health threat to the total community and may find themselves in conflict with law-enforcement agencies. For such reasons as these it is essential to make special efforts to understand the emotional and social conflicts which occur in contact situations, to devise ways to ease the transition for immigrant peoples, and to strive for greater understanding and sympathy from both modern medical practitioners and minority groups.

This book describes some of the conflicts in the relationships between Spanish-speaking people of Mexican descent in a California community and the English-speaking medical personnel with whom they have contact. Although contacts between English-speaking health workers and Spanish-speaking patients are usually friendly and rewarding, there are occasions when cultural differences lead to misunderstanding, skepticism, or fear. The following sketches will illustrate a few such cases. Although presented in seemingly fictional narration, they are in fact based on observed and recorded incidents.

A District nurse calls on a new mother.—"Why haven't you brought the baby into the clinic for his check-up, Lupe?" the district nurse asked a young Mexican-American mother. The baby was more than three months old and had not been seen by a doctor since the mother and child were discharged from the hospital maternity ward. The nurse was hot, tired, pressed for time, and mystified at her client's apparent lack of concern. Several clinic appointments had been broken without any explanation from Lupe. Flies buzzed about the kitchen, lighting on plates of uncovered food on the table. The nurse compressed her lips. "You really must get a screen on that back door—you can't have flies all over the baby." She walked to the iron bed standing in a corner of the kitchen and threw back the lace coverlet which covered the baby from head to toe. "Poor little fellow," she thought, "all covered up on such a hot day."

Later, after a somewhat reluctant mother had agreed to keep her appointment at the clinic the next week, the nurse said to me, "I just can't understand these people. The clinical facilities are available to them free of charge, but they won't take the trouble to bring the baby in for a routine examination. What's the matter with them?"

Lupe turned away from the door after the nurse finally left. She sighed and made the sign of the cross. "Thanks to God, that's over," she said to herself. She carried the baby, now crying from the disturbance of the nurse's examination, back to the bed, and carefully covered him again with the lace coverlet—a special gift from his godmother—to keep the flies away from him. She glanced at the gaping hole in the screen door which the landlord might never repair. She called the three older children in for lunch, which by this time was cold on the table. The oldest, Maria, would soon celebrate her *cumpleaños,* her fifth birthday. How could she get the baby to the clinic, she wondered. Her husband was picking fruit now—up at half-past five in the morning and never home until after dark. There was just nobody else this time of year to watch the children—everybody works during the fruit season. She would just have to take all the children with her. She would carry the baby, and the two older children could walk, but the twenty blocks to the clinic and home again would be hard for Pepito, not quite two. It seemed so silly—the baby was so fat and healthy. "What was the matter with that crazy nurse—couldn't she see that the baby didn't need a doctor?"

A medical social worker interviews a sanatorium patient.—The medical social worker was puzzled. He sat at his desk and thumbed through Tony's sanatorium records. There it was: "Antonio Prado, age thirty-seven, married, five living children, Mexican—active primary tuberculosis, moderately advanced, still unarrested." He had been admitted to the hospital just two months ago, and yet Tony kept begging, day after day, to go home now. With five children at home, Tony could not be released until his tuberculosis was fully arrested—it would be criminal negligence. He should have some consideration for his own children, if not for himself. The social worker turned to me. "That's one of my biggest problems," he said. "So many of them are like Tony; they keep asking me why they have to stay in the hospital when they feel so good now. And when I explain, they don't seem to comprehend. What can I say to make them understand?"

Antonio Prado left the social worker's office and started down the hall toward his ward. He knew the social worker was probably right—he shouldn't go home until the doctors said he was all right. But how could he be really sick when he felt so good—as strong as he had ever felt? He knew he could do a full day's work if they'd just let him go home. He couldn't hurt anybody, because they had told him just last week that he wasn't active any more; his test was negative. Antonio wished he could make them understand that he had to get out of the hospital to help his family. His wife had to work at the cannery long hours, and couldn't watch the kids. Now the oldest boy was in trouble with the juvenile authorities—he had gotten mixed up with some boys who had stolen a car. And Juan, the second son, wanted to quit school and go to work. Tony thought of his own life, of his childhood in Mexico, where a grade-school education had been considered good enough. Now here in California, Tony thought, he had spent the best years of his life as a day laborer, just because he didn't have enough education to do anything else. He didn't want that to happen to his sons, but it was going to happen if he didn't get out of the hospital pretty soon. How could he keep his sons in school and away from bad company when he was stuck here? That social worker was okay, Tony thought—*muy amable*, but he just didn't listen to Tony's problems. How could he make him understand?

A sick child is admitted to the hospital.—The doctor on emergency service at the county hospital was exhausted after a long night on duty: car-accident victims, stab wounds, acute appendicitis, and a half-dozen other emergencies. Armando Lopez and his son were next on the list. It took the doctor just a few minutes to realize that the boy was acutely ill with lobar pneumonia. He looked at Armando; yes, it was the same man who had already brought two other children to the hospital with pneumonia. The doctor's patience was at an end. "This is the third child you've brought in here in this condition within a week. If you were a good father and loved your children, you wouldn't let them get sick like this!" As the doctor turned to sign an order for admitting the child to the hospital, he said to the assisting nurse, "What's the matter with these people? Why do they wait until they're half dead before they come to the doctor? Then they blame us if we don't perform a miracle."

Armando frowned as he stood beside his sick son. He was sure he had understood the doctor: hadn't he said that he, Armando, was a bad father? After all, when the kids got sick and didn't get better even with the best *remedios* he could buy for them, he used his precious gasoline to drive the long miles from the ranch into town to the doctor. How could a man be a bad father when his children were always first in his thoughts? Armando remembered once before when the baby hadn't been able to sleep at night. That time Armando had brought the baby to the hospital, and the doctor had really bawled him out. The baby wasn't really sick, the doctor had said—don't take up the doctor's time with these silly things, he was told. And now, when he had waited until he knew the children were really sick, he was called a bad father. You can't win with these crazy *gringos*, Armando thought.

A doctor makes a house call.—The doctor had one more house call to make on the east side. He was greeted at the door by Mrs. Santiago, the daughter of the patient, Doña Isabel. Mrs. Santiago escorted him into a bedroom where the patient was, surrounded by a half-dozen relatives. She was a thin, wizened little woman, about seventy-five, eyes bright with fever. He approached her bed; and only with difficulty and with the help of her relatives was he able to perform his examination and administer a shot of penicillin. Throughout his examination, the patient kept muttering to her daughter in Spanish and looking daggers at the doctor. As he closed his bag and left the house, he laughed to himself. What a crazy little lady, he thought. She acted like I was about to poison her, instead of trying to help her. What do you suppose she was afraid of?

Doña Isabel was angry and frightened when the tall stranger with the black bag came into her room. Her daughter and son-in-law had lied to her again—they had promised not to send for the American doctor. She remembered well her grandson's first-born, the little *angelito* who had been killed by the American doctors. She had kept telling the family that the baby was *asustado*—sick with fright—and that he must be taken to the *curandera*—a woman who knew all the herbs and remedies for children. But they had taken the baby to the American doctor instead. It was to be expected when the baby died—and only because nobody would listen to her. In Jalisco she had seen many babies cured of this disease, but here in California the doctors didn't know how to cure such things.

Doña Isabel saw the doctor take out his instruments. She pulled the blankets up tight under her chin. "Make him leave me alone," she begged her daughter, but no one made a move to help her. Finally, trembling, she closed her eyes and placed her life in the hands of the Blessed Lady of Guadalupe.

Those who work with Spanish-speaking patients may recognize familiar problems in the above examples. Lupe, Tony, Armando, and Doña Isabel are not unusual people. In many ways they are typical of patients everywhere, of whatever ethnic or national background. In other respects they are uniquely Mexican-American in their attitudes and behavior.

Medical workers usually expect patients to behave in certain ways and are often puzzled when Spanish-speaking people fail to conform to those expectations. They ask, "Why won't they come in for routine examinations? What's the matter with them?" Or, "Why won't they stay in the hospital? How can I make them understand that they are ill? What are they afraid of?"

In the following chapters an attempt has been made to answer some of these questions by describing some aspects of the lives of Spanish-speaking people, their families and friends, their jobs, houses, religion, and community life. Out of an understanding of Mexican-Americans and their culture may come some solutions to their medical problems.

— 1

THE VALLEY, THE TOWN, AND THE PEOPLE

THIS BOOK deals with the Spanish-speaking people of San Jose, in the Santa Clara Valley of northern California.[1]

In the river valleys of northern California the soil is rich and fertile. Water from melting Sierra snows flows in many streams through the valleys to the Pacific; much is captured on its way and diverted into irrigation canals. Summer and winter the air is mild; over the Pacific slopes nature is kind to fields, orchards, and vineyards. From the first plump berries of early spring to the last golden fruit for Thanksgiving tables, the land yields a plentiful harvest.

At the southern tip of San Francisco Bay lies the Santa Clara

[1] For more details on the factual and historical material reported in this chapter, see Margaret Clark, Sickness and Health in *Sal si Puedes:* Mexican-Americans in a California Community. (Ph.D. dissertation) University of California, Berkeley, 1957.

The reader should note that Spanish words are italicized only the first time they are used. For the meanings of Spanish words, see the glossary.

7

Valley, a broad expanse of rich farmland. Its largest city, San Jose, centers on the Guadalupe River which flows northward to the bay. From San Jose the valley rises gently on the east to meet the grassy slopes of the Diablo Range. To the west and south rise the more distant Santa Cruz Mountains, with their forests of coastal redwood. On either side of the valley, mountain peaks rise to elevations of three to four thousand feet, but the valley itself lies almost at sea level. In greatest width, it is approximately twenty miles across and its length extends some sixty miles southeast from the salt marshes of the bay shore to the point where the plain narrows and vanishes into the mountains of San Benito County.

Although annual rainfall averages fifteen inches on the valley floor and as much as thirty inches in the surrounding foothills, most of the rain comes during the winter months. During spring and summer— the agricultural season—the skies are usually clear, the land arid, and fields and orchards must be irrigated. In winter and early spring the rivers and creeks in the bordering mountains swell, and water is dammed and held in many reservoirs along the rim of the valley, to be released into irrigation channels when it is needed. The main watercourses are the Coyote and Guadalupe rivers and their tributaries. Additional water for irrigation comes from artesian wells, which produce water from depths of from 50 to 250 feet in most parts of the valley.

Fertile soil, mild climate, and abundant water make the valley a rich garden, whose growing season extends from 254 days at San Jose to 316 days at Los Gatos in the western foothills [45]. In the early days of European settlement, the chief crops of the region were wheat and corn; but since 1900, grains have largely been replaced by strawberries, cherries, apricots, green beans and peas, pears, prunes, wine grapes, walnuts, tomatoes, and an almost unlimited variety of garden vegetables.

Since more than 88 per cent of the total acreage of the valley is farmland, most industry in towns and cities is understandably dependent on agriculture [45]. Food processing accounts for much of the industrial activity: the towns teem with canneries, fruit and vegetable packing houses, fruit-drying establishments, frozen-food plants, and wineries. Other industries based on agriculture produce such items as irrigation pumps and chemical fertilizers. Nonagricultural industry includes steel, cement, and electrical-machinery production and automobile assembly.

Observation of new building and development in the valley reveals that the land use is changing. Orchards and fields in many localities are giving way to suburban residential tracts. Farms and pastures have been transformed into housing subdivisions occupied by urban workers who commute to their jobs in factories and offices in San Francisco and the East Bay cities. Perhaps the whole face of the valley will soon be changed. But in 1956, the passing of time in the land is still marked by planting, fruition, and harvest; and on the bounty of the harvest rest the fortunes of the valley people.

San Jose, the seat of Santa Clara County, is the economic and population center of the valley. In 1950 its population was just over 100,000, and in 1955 approximately 150,000 [42].

The history of the city dates back to 1777, when a pueblo was established on the banks of the Guadalupe River four miles south of the Mission of Santa Clara. The settlement was formed at the suggestion of Don Felipe Neve, then Spanish governor of California, and by order of King Charles III of Spain. Its first occupants were fourteen men skilled in agriculture: five civilians, and nine soldiers from the garrison of the Presidio of San Francisco. The express purpose of the settlement was to put into cultivation a tract of land in the Santa Clara Valley in order to provide grain and vegetables for both the mission and the military post at San Francisco [24].

Although San Jose was first a Spanish and later a Mexican pueblo, American settlers began to arrive and establish homes in the area as early as 1830. Relatively large numbers of Americans continued to immigrate to San Jose throughout the years preceding the acquisition of California by the United States. Metamorphosis of the pueblo into an American town was rapid. A city directory of San Jose and its surrounding area published in 1876, just thirty years after the fall of the Mexican government in California, contains only five Spanish names. Of these, three were listed as natives of Mexico, one of California, and one of Spain [46]. Of the five, only two were listed as owning land in the county.

Although there may have been people living in or near San Jose whose names were not included in the records, it is abundantly clear that there was only a handful of Spanish-speaking people left in

1876. Yet, by 1955, the picture had again changed radically. Of the 425,000 people living in Santa Clara County in 1955, approximately one out of eight was a Spanish-speaking person of Mexican descent [9]. This group now constitutes one of the largest concentrations of Mexican-Americans in California. Only Los Angeles, Alameda, and San Bernardino counties have Spanish-speaking populations that are larger [50].

What brought so many Spanish-speaking people into the valley? When did they arrive and where did they come from? Many of the subjects of this study told us of their coming to San Jose. The following stories are representative.

Juana was born on a ranch near Phoenix, Arizona, in 1915. Her parents had left their home village near Hermosillo, Sonora, in Mexico, in 1910. They left home and relatives behind because there was no money and no work, and because they had heard stories about jobs paying good wages to be found across the border. The young couple made their way northward, and crossed the border on foot near Nogales, carrying on their backs what few possessions they had. Juana's father found work first in the copper mines in northern Arizona. He worked as a miner for four years, but his health failed and he moved his family to Phoenix, where he got work as a farm laborer, a job which gave him the sunshine and fresh air he needed. There Juana was born. When she was only a few years old, her family moved to Utah, where her father worked on a railroad section gang. When the railroad was completed, Juana's parents once more moved on in search of work. They heard that people were needed to dig potatoes in Idaho, and it was in the potato fields that Juana first met her husband, Marcos.

Marcos, like Juana's parents, was born in Mexico in the State of Michoacán. He had come to the United States only a few years before he met Juana, immigrating to Oregon when he was eighteen years old, to work for the railroad. Later he worked there as a logger before moving to Utah. After Marcos and Juana were married, they and Juana's family moved to California to get work in the fruit orchards. They first came to Brawley, then to Fresno, then to Sacramento, and finally in 1949 to San Jose. Marcos has had steady work as a foreman for a prune grower for the past five years. All of their five children were born in California.

Pío, who runs a small business in San Jose, was born in Torreón, in the State of Coahuila, Mexico. When he was only a few months old, his parents emigrated to a Texas border town. In Mexico, Pío's father had made a comfortable living for his family as a harness maker. However, the Mexican Revolution of 1910 with its following years of discord made life difficult for a peace-loving craftsman, so in 1915 he took his small savings and, with his wife and infant son, traveled northward across the Rio Grande into Texas. From 1915 until 1923, he worked as a harness maker, but with the coming of the automobile there was less and less demand for his skill. Finally, he decided to move once again, this time to California. The family came first to Salinas in 1923, where Pío's father found work in the lettuce fields. Each summer the whole family would come north to San Jose to pick prunes, camping in a tent near the orchards. In 1926, Pío's father bought a small lot just outside San Jose and, with the help of his sons and some of his friends, built a small house for his family. Pío's parents have since died, but he and his wife and children still live in the same house on the outskirts of town.

Edmundo was nine years old when he came to the United States. He was brought to California by his parents in 1916. In the years before the Mexican Revolution, his father had operated a dry-goods store in a town in the State of Jalisco, Mexico. Edmundo's father was a successful merchant and was able to accumulate a small amount of property, including a farm near Guadalajara. But he was known as an antirevolutionary, and in 1916 his store and house were burned and his property confiscated. In fear of his life, he took his family and what money he had and fled across the California border. At that time Los Angeles was engaged in paving its streets, so Edmundo's father and older brothers went to work for the city, laboring with pick and shovel and moving earth with mule-drawn graders. Edmundo went through high school in Los Angeles and got his first job as a construction worker in the San Fernando Valley. In Los Angeles, too, he met his wife, who had been born in southern Colorado. Edmundo decided that he would study bookkeeping at night and try to get a better-paying job. By 1946, he had saved enough capital to move his family to San Jose and to open a small business of his own. Edmundo's three sons were all born in San Jose. The family, including Edmundo's aged parents, lives in a new home in an east San Jose suburb.

The stories of Juana, Marcos, Pío, and Edmundo are typical of those of the subjects of this study, but there are many exceptions to the patterns of residence which they exemplify. One of Pío's neighbors, for example, comes from an old California family. He knows that his grandfather was born in Santa Clara County, near the town of Milpitas, and that his great-grandfather owned land in the Calaveras Canyon approximately twelve miles northwest of San Jose; but where his great-grandfather was born, he does not know. Others are more recent arrivals from Mexico, having entered the United States within the past ten years. Most of the Spanish-speaking people in San Jose, however, were either born in the United States or have lived in this country for more than twenty-five years.

Although Mexican-American families live in scattered areas throughout the county, there are a dozen or more communities in and near town and cities whose residents are predominantly Spanish-speaking people. One such community, which is the locale of this study, is an unincorporated suburban area adjacent to the eastern boundary of San Jose. The community is sometimes known as the Mayfair District.

The population of Mayfair is approximately 4,500 persons, of whom about two-thirds, or 3,000 people, are of Mexican descent. The district covers an area of approximately one and one-third square miles, a roughly rectangular tract three-fourths miles wide and one and three-fourths miles long. About one-third of the land is in cultivation, the remaining two-thirds being subdivided into residential tracts.

Mayfair is bounded on the west by U. S. Highway 101, a superhighway which runs southward from San Francisco through the Santa Clara Valley and on to Los Angeles. On the north it is delimited by Alum Rock Road, a main thoroughfare connecting the city of San Jose with the eastern foothills. Toward the east and south, the residential area borders on open farmland and pasture. Silver Creek, a tributary of the Coyote River, runs from east to west through the area. During the summer months Silver Creek is a dry arroyo, and the children of Mayfair often play on its steep banks or in the dry sand of the creek bed.

The area which is now Mayfair was, in the days of the Spanish and Mexican settlement of San Jose, a part of the town's *ejido*, or "common"—publicly owned, uncultivated land adjacent to the settled area. The ejido was not appropriated to a single individual, but was used for grazing, firewood gathering, and the like, by all residents. It was also designed to "adorn the entrance of the place" and provide for proper "ventilation" [24].

After 1846, when the Pueblo of San Jose was surrendered to American authorities, large sectors of municipal lands were granted to individuals by the newly formed town council. The present Mayfair area, however, was not included in any of those grants, but was a part of the pueblo tracts which were conveyed to a city board of commissioners in 1858 to be sold to private owners and the proceeds used to pay municipal debts [24].

A map of east San Jose published in 1876 shows that all the Mayfair land had been sold to private owners, and was divided among twelve landholders, the size of the estates ranging from 10 to 285 acres. In 1896, the first subdivision of land into house lots was made, but very few houses were built in Mayfair until about 1914, when a number of Puerto Ricans began to move into San Jose. By 1927, about fifteen families had settled in Mayfair. During the following year Mexican immigrants began to come into the community; some of them bought lots and built houses; others camped near the settlement during the agricultural season, living in tents and working in nearby fields and orchards.

Over the years the character of the community has changed. Many other subdivisions have been established; tents have long since disappeared and given way to permanent housing; schools and churches have been built; and approximately 3,000 Spanish-speaking people now occupy the land. Among these people are Armando, Doña Isabel, and Pío. Mayfair is their home.

— 2

THE PATTERN OF COMMUNITY LIFE

SHOULD SOMEONE ask Armando what group of people he belongs to, he might be frankly puzzled. Armando has not thought much about being a member of a social group. A number of responses might occur to him: "I'm a Mexican," or "I'm an American, like you," or "I live in east San Jose," or "I was born in Texas." He might think about his occupation and say, "I'm a member of the Teamsters' Union." His religious affiliation might first come to mind, and Armando would answer with the name of his church. He might think, "I'm a member of the Gutierrez family," or "I'm from the Sunset Street neighborhood," or "I belong to the American Legion." To Armando, all these are correct answers to the question, "Where do you belong?"

Public health workers are interested in Armando's place in community life because the social groups to which he belongs determine so much of what he believes, fears, trusts, ignores, or is concerned about in matters which influence his health and the health of his family and friends. In order to reach Armando with information about disease and its control, it is imperative to know the channels through which he receives information. In order to influence Armando's beliefs on health, it is important to know whose word he trusts, what leaders he follows, and which groups he is influenced by.

In the following pages we will talk about some of the social groupings of the subjects of this study, the functions of those groups, their characteristics, and their influence on the lives of the people who compose them.

A Mexican-American resident of east San Jose may be thought of as a member of three sorts of extended social groupings, comparable to a series of ever-widening circles. These three are: (1) a *barrio* or ward, a spatially defined unit roughly equivalent to "neighborhoods" in American towns and cities; (2) a larger community composed of several barrios, the Mayfair District; and (3) a still larger San Jose Mexican-American colony, of which Mayfair is but one segment.

THE COLONY

Armando and his neighbors often speak of themselves as members of the *colonia*, or San Jose Mexican-American colony. It is composed of groups of Spanish-speaking families of Mexican ancestry who live scattered throughout the urban and suburban San Jose area. Members of the colony, like Mexican-Americans in the Southwest, are not easily distinguished from the rest of the population of San Jose by any single criterion. For example, several distinct dialects of Spanish are spoken in Mexican-American homes (see chap. 3), and the use of English may be either negligible or extensive. The people differ in educational level, citizenship, wealth, complexion, and religious conviction. Some fear outsiders and trust only those within the colony, whereas others seek English-speaking associates and claim little kinship with others of Mexican descent. Some of the people live only for a dream of returning to Mexico; to others, Mexico is a foreign place of little interest which they have never seen.

In spite of the heterogeneity of the Mexican-Americans, Saunders [43] has claimed that

Viewed as a group, they do have characteristics that distinguish them from the Anglo population. Physically, they are easily identifiable because of their common, but by no means uniform, genetic inheritance from the populations of sixteenth- and seventeenth-century Spain and various North American Indian tribal groups. Socially, they possess a variety of combinations of cultural traits that can be traced to Spain or Mexico and that are not generally shared by Anglos. Psychologically, they tend to identify themselves as members of a distinct group and to be so identified by Anglos.

FACTORS IN SOCIAL CLEAVAGE

It is clear to observers of San Jose Mexican-American society that, although there are factors which tend to divide the community into smaller fragments, other forces create a sense of kinship which unifies the community. The colony is host to opposing forces, some disruptive and others integrative.

Social Classes

Although social classes are poorly defined in the San Jose colonia, Spanish-speaking people recognize class differences. "My people can't seem to coöperate with each other," one Mayfair merchant complained; "They won't associate with people who are below them, and they are jealous and resentful of those who are above them."

Paula, the wife of a construction foreman, classifies members of the colony into four groups: the lowest social class, the *braceros* (Mexican nationals imported for farm labor during the harvest season), are actually outsiders, she feels. They are single men who have no family ties or other obligations to the community and therefore "don't really belong" to the colony. Mexican-Americans generally express feelings of hostility and resentment toward braceros. Some typical comments about them are: "They come in and take jobs away from our own people, because they work for almost nothing; the braceros get the jobs and our people have to go on relief." "The Nationals are a real menace to society—they bring in diseases from Mexico." "The braceros aren't like the rest of us who came to California to make homes: they don't care about the community—they get drunk and get into fights and give the Mexican people a bad name." "The braceros usually come from the country; they are *campesinos, indios,* and *tontos* who are pretty ignorant.[1] They don't

---

[1] "*Campesinos, indios,* and *tontos*" may be translated roughly: "rustics, Indians, and stupid people." *Tonto* (foolish, stupid) is often intended to imply the same meaning as the American terms, "country hick" or "hillbilly."

know very much, and can't get along very well here in the United States."

Paula identifies the rest of the Spanish-speaking community as comprising three social grades: (1) *la alta sociedad,* or "high society"; (2) *los medianos,* the middle class; and (3) *los de abajo,* the "lowly ones."

Paula, who spent her childhood years in Mexico, says that she and her family are medianos now. When her family first came from Mexico to California, though, their estate was not so exalted. "When I was a young girl in Mexico," she reminisced, "we were real poor; my father was dead and my mother had to take work as a maid for a family in Chihuahua." Paula recalled that her mother's wages were three pesos a month, plus food and shelter for herself and her six children. "Often we were *descalzos,* barefooted, and I can remember the first time I ever ate with a knife and fork instead of my fingers. When I was sixteen years old, we came to the United States, and my mother got a job that paid twenty-five dollars a month. To us that seemed like a lot of money. We were still poor, but here we could at least have shoes and things like knives and forks."

"Often I have thought of going back to Mexico," Paula said, "but in Mexico we would always have been los de abajo. I've figured out that it's good for the poor to leave Mexico and come to the United States; sure, you can be poor right here in San Jose, but never as poor as you could be in Mexico."

Paula has pretty clear ideas about what establishes people as los de abajo: "They usually move around, following the crops, don't have steady jobs, and never have quite enough food or clothes. During hard times when there is no fruit to be picked, they have to 'go on the county' [seek public assistance]." Although Paula and her neighbors regard migrant workers as their social inferiors, the medianos feel a sympathy for and kinship with this group that does not characterize their attitudes toward braceros. Of los de abajo, a Spanish-speaking clerk said, "I really get mad at some of my people who look down on poor people and think they are superior to them; most of us were pretty poor ourselves when we first came to San Jose. They think that poor people are stupid, but that's not true."

Paula has mixed feelings about la alta sociedad, the "high society" Mexican-Americans. On the one hand, she admires and envies

Spanish-speaking people who have higher incomes, better houses, more education, and more prestige in the colony. "Juan Campa is a big man in this town," she said. "He is someone the Mexican people can be proud of, and he has done a lot to help our people." On the other hand, Paula feels that many of the more "successful" Mexican-Americans in San Jose are traitors to their own people, disassociate themselves from other Spanish-speaking groups, and ally themselves with Anglos. "The big shots don't live in the same neighborhoods with us," she remarked. "Even if they once lived here, when they've made enough money, they usually move into town or to one of the fashionable suburbs like Cupertino or Saratoga." The alta sociedad Mexican-Americans, Paula said, move into Anglo neighborhoods and start speaking English most of the time. "Some of their children pretend not to be able to speak Spanish because they are ashamed of being Mexican. Sometimes they won't have anything more to do with their old friends, and sometimes pretend not to be Mexican anymore; they say they are 'Spanish-Americans.' They don't mix with lower-class Mexicans, but just with their own kind." The members of the colony whom Paula considers "upper class" are those who live in expensive houses, have professional or white-collar jobs, go to Anglo churches, and join Anglo organizations. Paula feels that many of the "upper crust" have acquired prosperity not through hard work or frugality, but simply because "they were lucky—they got the breaks." She attributes the high social and economic status of "high society" Mexican-Americans to chance rather than to industry or intelligence.

Paula and her neighbors are glad that they are not poor, but they also disclaim a desire for wealth. "Of course, we might wish we had more money, but in some ways we're glad we aren't rich. Rich people have to spend all their time worrying about their money and how to keep from losing it. It's not good to be too rich, but it's worse to be too poor. The best way is to have a steady job and make enough money to live on. That way you don't have to worry about anything and you can really be happy." Paula spoke for many of the people of Mayfair when she said, "It's not a bad thing to be a mediano; each day we live life and each night we sleep sound."

The Spanish-speaking community takes on different aspects as seen through the eyes of the "successful" Mexican-American in San Jose. An American-born businessman, classified as "alta sociedad" by the medianos, acknowledged only two social classes within the colony. "There are a lot of us who are trying to get ahead and make a decent life for our children," he said, "but most of the people just don't seem to care. Most of the people in Mayfair are pretty low class; they are lazy and don't care how they live. That place is really a slum, and the Mexican people ought to be ashamed of it."

More prosperous members of the community claim that they can be distinguished from lower-class people by the fact that they are better dressed, have more polite manners, speak better Spanish and English, and value education for themselves and their children. "We see to it that our children get a good education," one informant claimed, "but lower-class people take their kids out of school and put them to work as soon as they can earn a dime." Higher-class individuals also believe that poor people are more resentful of Anglos and feel inferior to them.

A Spanish-speaking professional man commented that well-to-do Mexican-Americans feel one of two ways about poorer members of the colony: "Some of my friends feel responsible for needy people in the community and try to help as much as they can. A man might work in a service organization, contribute to charities, or support the Mexican labor movement. Other people in town who have acquired a little security themselves want to have no connection with poorer Spanish-speaking families; in fact, they don't even want to be called Mexicans themselves or be associated with their own people."

The "higher-class" members' description of the colony's class structure is similar to the view of Mexican-American society held by the San Jose Anglos, who for the most part refer to Spanish-speaking people as either "low class" or "high class." Since the subjects of this study are the people of Mayfair, that is, los medianos, the class structure of the colony will be described in these pages from their point of view.

In addition to the criteria of income and standard of living, colony members consider occupation, speech, education, property ownership, and other factors when identifying people with one or another of the social classes. Class distinction is not an incidental or inconsequential pattern in the life of Spanish-speaking San Jose—it is a main strand woven into the fabric of community life. It helps erect some of the invisible barriers which divide the people and prevent effective cooperation of the Mexican-American colony as a whole.

The implications of class structure for health programs are discussed in the final chapter of this book. Health-program planners will have to contend with the fact that class differentiation in Mexican-American society poses real problems of indigenous leadership. "High-class" Mexican-American "leaders" who work and communicate well with Anglos may be rejected as leaders by medianos, or families of lower socioeconomic class. Problems may also be raised by the fact that better-educated or wealthier Mexican-Americans who have leadership ability may divorce themselves from the Spanish-speaking group and be unwilling to work closely with fellow colonists in community health and welfare programs.

Mexicans or Americans?

Nearly 80 per cent of the Spanish-speaking people of San Jose are native Americans. Most American-born persons, however, are under twenty-five years of age. The adult population of the colony is more equally divided into native and foreign-born residents. Difference in place of birth is reflected in conflicting national loyalties.

Most of those born north of the border understandably consider themselves Americans and usually express pride in their place of birth. They believe that the abundant life for themselves and for their people is to be found in the "American way of life." Many of them dream of and work toward the day when Mexican-Americans will become fully integrated into American society at large.

It is sometimes difficult for those born and reared in this country to understand the reluctance of many Mexican immigrants to disclaim their citizenship, national loyalties, mother tongue, and native traditions in favor of those of the United States. "There are a lot of Mexican people," one native Californian observed, "who came to the United States years ago but have never accepted the idea that this is their country now. They don't apply for American citizenship and don't try to learn English because they kid themselves that they are living here temporarily; some of them have been here 'temporarily' for thirty or forty years!"

The decision to seek United States citizenship is a difficult one for patriotic Mexicans to make. One naturalized American said, "People who were born and reared in Mexico continue to have the hearts of patriots and many believe that if they become American citizens they are traitors to Mexico. Some of the people even have the idea that when someone becomes a United States citizen, he is required to trample on the Mexican flag."

The dream of some day returning to Mexico is shared by many expatriates in San Jose. Although many have not seen their homeland for thirty years or more, they keep their memories of the old country alive in reminiscences, legends, stories, and songs. "My mother never stopped telling us about the old days in Mexico," one woman reported. "She never tired of telling us stories of her native village in Guanajuato; she never let us children forget the things that her village was noted for, its handicrafts and arts, its songs and its stories about the 'big men' in the village and their accomplishments. She made it all sound so beautiful with her descriptions of the mountains and the lakes, the old traditions, the happy people, and the dances and weddings and fiestas. From the time I was a small child I always wanted to go back to Mexico and see the village where my mother was born."

"But all these dreams of going back to Mexico," she continued, "never came true for my family. My parents always said that soon we would go back. But years and years went by, and soon they were old. We children grew up and married and had families of our own. After that, it was too late for them to go back—their roots were here in California, and all their old friends and relatives in Mexico were dead. There was nothing to go back to, so they stayed on in the United States."

In the minds of the Spanish-speaking people of San Jose there are two conceptions of the colonia: some visualize it as a group of loyal Mexicans and their children and grandchildren, who for various reasons have not been able to return to their own country; others see the colony as an American ethnic community of Mexican origin which, like Italian, Irish, or Scandinavian immigrant groups, will eventually be absorbed into the pattern of American life. These contrasting images are reflected in the more structured aspects of community life. There are in San Jose formal organizations which are "Americanist" in their stated aims. (Examples of "Americanist" groups are: the San Jose chapter of the state-wide Community Service Organization; the Civic Co-ordinating Council, a local group; the Clifford Rodriguez Post of the American Legion; and the United Latin-Americans of America.) These organizations have programs aimed at integration of the Spanish-speaking colony into Anglo society. Their goals for Mexican-Americans are American citizenship, wider and more effective knowledge of the English language, and full participation in the civic, political, and economic affairs of San Jose. The "Americanist" groups contrast with another organization (Comisión Honorífica Mexicana, or Mexican Honorific Commission) which is sponsored by the Mexican consul in San Francisco. As a "nationalistic" association, its members oppose the recruitment of Mexican nationals to become United States citizens and attempt instead to preserve the essentially "Mexican" character of the colony.

People are divided in their support of the opposing organizations. During the year in which this study was conducted, disagreement between contending organizations led to a division of the community into two rival factions. Conflicting national loyalties, then, is an additional factor promoting disunion within the Mexican-American community.

Sects and Other Social Segments

Religious activities are a large and prominent part of the panorama of life for many people of the colony. According to one estimate,[2] only 4 per cent of Spanish-speaking residents of San Jose have no church affiliation. Of the remaining 96 per cent, an estimated 70 per cent are Catholic and 26 per cent are Protestant. Catholics attend mass at several churches in the San Jose area, three of which have Spanish-speaking priests.[3] The Protestant group is subdivided into various denominations, most of which are "fundamentalist" or "revivalist" in character.

Although there is no open hostility between members of the various religious sects in the community, members of one sect tend to limit their social relationships to those with people of similar religious preference. This is particularly true of some of the independent Protestant congregations, whose members often have close friendly

---

[2] These figures are based on a 20 per cent sample of Spanish-speaking persons of Mexican descent who registered for a Mayfair District chest X-ray survey in November, 1955. About one thousand persons were sampled—roughly one-third of the Mexican-American community.

[3] The majority of Catholics in Mayfair attend the Chapel of Our Lady of Guadalupe, near Mayfair Elementary School; other churches, outside Mayfair, which especially attract Spanish-speaking parishioners are the Church of the Holy Family, St. Joseph's Church (both of which have occasional sermons in Spanish), and the Church of the Five Wounds, which has a Lisbon-born priest who delivers sermons in Portuguese.

relations only with fellow parishioners. A certain provincialism typifies the attitudes of members of one religious sect toward "outsiders."

Other factors operate to subdivide the Mexican-American colony into smaller and smaller segments. One of these is the fact that the people have come to San Jose from all parts of the American Southwest and from different regions of Mexico. Families who formerly lived in the Texas border area, for example, seek out others from the same locality. A group of such families from Texas or Colorado or Coahuila or Michoacán may form a clique within a single neighborhood and establish close relationships primarily with members of that clique. Marta, a thirty-six-year-old woman from a Texas border community, has a circle of close friends who have come to San Jose from the same region. "It really makes me mad," she complained, "when I have to be around that Mrs. Valdéz [a neighbor of hers originally from northern New Mexico]. She always talks about people from Texas, and says that all Texans are no good. I tell her that Texans are as good as anybody from New Mexico—maybe better. She has her own friends, and she can stick with them; I don't ever invite her to my house any more."

Not many people are as articulate as Marta in expressing preference for those from their own home locality. One more frequently hears comments of this sort: "Whenever my car breaks down, I take it to Manuel's garage; I can trust him, because he's from Jalisco, like me."

Age Groups

"There's one thing that we've learned in trying to form successful organizations among our people," a civic-minded Mexican-American said. "You can't mix young and old people together in an organization; they're just not interested in the same things. If you plan activities for one age-group, the other completely loses interest. Here in San Jose, there's a big difference between a man of thirty and a man of forty-five. They don't want the same things—they don't even think alike."

The tendency of people to group themselves into age grades is one which is familiar to members of Anglo-American society as well. But even though differences in age groups are present in Anglo communities, they are seen in exaggerated form within the San Jose colony. The role that immigration and culture change has played in widening social distance between different generations of Mexican-Americans will be discussed in chapter 6.

We have seen that the people of the colony are a heterogeneous group. Within their ranks are those who are prosperous and those who are poor; there are ignorant and learned, native and foreign born, citizens and noncitizens, the very young and the very old. In planning health programs for Spanish-speaking communities, this heterogeneity should be borne in mind.

FACTORS IN SOCIAL COHESION

For all the influences which erect social barriers between members of the colonia, Mexican-Americans feel a strong sense of kinship with each other, in contrast with their feeling of separation from the English-speaking majority. They frequently use terms such as "our community," "we people," "those of our race," or "we Mexicans." When a Spanish-speaking citizen of San Jose needs legal advice, he is likely to consult a Spanish-speaking lawyer. He probably will have his automobile repaired by a Mexican-American mechanic or buy real estate through a broker within the colony. One member of the colony stated with confidence that a new appliance delivered to his home in damaged condition would be repaired by the store "because one of the delivery men said they would, and he's a Mexican."

In some respects the colony is like a family of brothers and sisters who may argue, fight, and compete among themselves, but in times of stress or in relations with outsiders stand together as a unit, offering each other trust and support. There are some powerful forces that foster community spirit.

Language

Many San Jose Mexican-Americans are bilingual, having learned Spanish first as children in their homes and English in the early years of elementary schooling. There are some, however, who speak only Spanish and others who speak English only with much difficulty. San Jose Mexican-Americans showed a marked preference for Spanish, and many who seemed reticent and withdrawn during a conversation in English became relaxed and articulate when expressing themselves in Spanish.

Adolescents and young adults ordinarily feel more at ease with English speakers than do their elders. Some of the younger people speak English whenever possible and try to encourage their parents, too, to use more English. But as of 1955 the language of the colony was still Spanish, and its common use helped to draw Mexican-Americans together into a unified group. For a fuller discussion of language, see chapter 3.

Common Channels of Communication

The existence of Spanish-language radio and press is an indication of language preference in the colony. There are three radio stations in San Jose which present Spanish-language broadcasts during a part of every day. Their Spanish-speaking announcers, who serve as disc jockeys, news reporters, and commercial announcers, are among the best-known personalities in the colony. Programs of recorded Mexican music are popular with radio listeners, and the voices of Mexican vocalists are as well-recognized in Spanish-speaking homes as the voices of the popular American singers are in Anglo households.

Almost as popular as musical programs are broadcasts in Spanish of world and local news. For some of the members of the colony who read neither American nor Mexican papers, Spanish-language news broadcasts are the prime source of information about national and international affairs. News reports cover not only leading stories from American wire services but also information of special interest to Mexican-Americans. Mexican political happenings, sports events involving Spanish-speaking athletes, and disasters such as earthquakes in Jalisco or floods in Acapulco are given special coverage. News of Spanish-speaking communities in other parts of the state is broadcast, the stories usually being taken from *La Opinion,* a Los Angeles Spanish-language daily paper. Items of interest in the local colony are collected by radio reporters themselves and passed on to the Spanish-speaking audience.

Similar methods of news gathering are used by two San Jose Spanish-language periodicals, a semimonthly tabloid and a weekly newspaper, both of which are widely circulated among members of the colony.[4] Copies of *La Opinion* are sold in several of the larger

[4] *El Excéntrico,* founded in 1950, is published semimonthly and distributed at no charge to Spanish-speaking readers through Mexican-American business establishments. Primarily a shopping guide and advertising journal, it also contains news of social events in the colony, such as birth and wedding announcements and reports of club activities. A weekly paper, *Eco Latino,* began publication early in 1955.

Mexican grocery and drug stores in San Jose. The supply is always exhausted soon after the papers are put on sale each day.

The Spanish-language radio and press in San Jose serve a need in mass communications which is not filled by any of the English-language media. The two English newspapers of the city (*The San Jose News* and *The San Jose Mercury*) either give scanty coverage or make no mention at all of events which are of great interest to Mexican-Americans. During the summer of 1955, for example, an entire Mexican-American family, six persons in all, drowned in a river near San Jose. One of the local Anglo papers made no mention of the incident at all, and the other one gave the story two inches in a back-page column. This disaster was the main topic of conversation among members of the colony for several days, and when the Spanish-language weekly paper came out with full front-page coverage of the incident, copies were sold almost as soon as they were put on the newsstands.

Many leaders in the colony feel that the Spanish-speaking community gets very poor publicity in the local Anglo press. The few news items which do appear about the Mexican-American community frequently deal with criminal acts, juvenile delinquency, substandard housing, and other social problems, or reports of disputes within the colony. Some examples of headlines for stories about the Spanish-speaking community which appeared in San Jose papers from 1952 to 1955 are: "Mexican-U. S. Group Denies Disunity"; "Mexican Community Feud in Eruption"; "Cockfight Pair Fined $100 Each"; "Mother of 3 Charged with $2,000 Fraud"; "East Side Vote Fraud Try Denied." During the same period there was some coverage of the more "positive" aspects of Mexican-American life, as indicated by the following headlines: "Legion Post Honors Barber for Helping Others Gain Citizenship"; "Spanish-speaking Women in Red Cross Drive"; "Mexican Parade, Fiesta Today"; "15,000 See Mexican Liberation Parade." During the thirteen months of research for this book, fewer than twenty newspaper articles appeared in the Anglo press dealing with the "positive" aspects of Mexican-American life. The achievements of Mexican-American civic groups, advances in adult education and citizenship programs among the people, and the

---

It contains local news of interest to the colony, social news, reviews of Mexican films, and features. Feature articles in 1955 included a series on major events and personalities in Mexican history.

activities of Spanish-speaking youth groups in the city were all largely unpublicized. Yet one out of seven San Jose citizens is a person of Mexican descent.

Reliance on their own channels of communication for news of the community, city, state, and world tends to separate the members of the colony from the Anglo community and to draw them into a closer-knit social unit.

If health information is to reach a large Spanish-speaking audience through mass media, Spanish-language media should be included. As a rule, information distributed through Spanish-language press and radio is more likely to find its way into neighborhood "grapevines" than is material appearing in the English media.

Kinship

Family connections are the most important social ties among people of the colony. Great emphasis is placed on kinship by blood or marriage, and people try to establish homes in neighborhoods where other relatives live. Paula, for example, has so many relatives living in San Jose that she has difficulty enumerating them all: her mother, four sisters and their husbands, thirty-three nieces and nephews, their twenty-four children, two aunts, five first cousins, seventeen second cousins, Paula's husband, their own four children, and her husband's many relatives—all are members of the colony.

In San Jose, as in other California Spanish-speaking communities, "grandparents, uncles, aunts, and cousins are considered part of the intimate family circle . . . they visit back and forth frequently; they form a common council in crisis or times of decision; they furnish mutual aid and provide a bulwark of interlocked strength for the individual" [48].

The family circle is widened still more among Mexican-Americans of Catholic faith by the institution of *compadrazgo,* a system which creates special ceremonial bonds between a child's parents and godparents. *Compadres* are often as intimate as brothers and sisters; their help is sought in troubled times; their advice is requested in making important decisions. "In some ways," a San Jose man said, "a compadre is better than a brother—he always respects you, always defends your honor and your reputation, and will always help you out of a jam."

The threads of kinship by blood, marriage, and compadrazgo

weave a strong network of relationships which supports the individual in the community and binds him to a large segment of the colony. An Anglo may walk the streets of San Jose as a lonely man among strangers; his Spanish-speaking neighbor walks the same streets but sees the faces of his brothers and compadres among the crowd.

For a fuller discussion of family life, including compadrazgo, see chapter 6.

Organizations

Paula's social relationships extend beyond her contacts with relatives and compadres because of her participation in the activities of formal organizations in the colony. She attends church at the Chapel of Our Lady of Guadalupe in east San Jose, and is a member of its Altar Society, the Sociedad Guadalupana. Paula likes working for the Altar Society, helping cook Mexican delicacies for the Sunday food sales at the church, taking part in the *jamaicas*, or church bazaars, which are held twice a year. She has made many friends among the other women of the Sociedad, and often visits with them in their homes to discuss the affairs of the church.

Paula also takes an interest in the Community Service Organization, a civic group which has helped many Mexicans to become American citizens and to register as voters. She is not naïve about Mexican-American civic groups—she has seen many of them organized only to die from lack of community support, divided leadership, or simply from flagging interest among their members. Paula is a little skeptical about "civic improvement leagues" until they have proved their worth to the colony in ways that she can understand and appreciate. "Most of the officers of the Community Service Organization are 'big shots,'" Paula said. "You have to wait for a while until you find out just what they're up to. But they did help us to get our streets paved in Mayfair, so they may not be so bad. We'll just have to wait and see." Paula does not attend meetings regularly, because she has too many responsibilities to her family and to her church. But she and her husband sometimes go to meetings "just to see what's going on." There she sometimes meets people from other parts of the colony whom she otherwise would never have known.

Paula and her mother became members of a *funeraria*, or "burial society," through buying life insurance policies from a Mexican-American insurance cooperative. Paula sometimes attends monthly membership meetings, where she becomes acquainted with fellow members. When someone in the funeraria dies, Paula, who is a devout Catholic, almost always attends the wake and the funeral, even though the deceased member may be Protestant. She feels it her duty to give comfort and support to the sorrowing family. The funeraria cuts across sectarian lines, linking Protestant and Catholic communities by bonds of sympathy during times of bereavement.

Although Paula has little time for other organizations, her life is affected by other formal groups supported by her relatives. Her husband is an officer in a Mexican-American credit union sponsored by the church; her brother is active in the Spanish-speaking American Legion Post in San Jose; her oldest daughter belongs to a Mexican-American youth club; her brother-in-law is a Knight of Columbus. Although Paula says, "I'm no joiner—I just stay at home and take care of my family," in hundreds of ways her daily life is knitted into the pattern of colony living by organized groupings of Spanish-speaking people.

Special Events and Recreation

To the casual Anglo observer, the most conspicuous factors in unification of the colony are the various public gatherings of Spanish-speaking people: the parades and fiestas which mark the celebration of Mexican national holidays on the fifth of May and the sixteenth of September; the big *bailes*, or public dances, at Mexican-American ballrooms, with music furnished by famous Latin-American orchestras; the boxing and the wrestling matches which feature Spanish-speaking athletes; the crowds of Mexican-American people who attend theaters which show Mexican films.

The whole colony turns out en masse to celebrate the *fiestas patrias*, the Mexican national holidays. For weeks before the festive day arrives, a wave of excitement runs through the community. There is much talk at Paula's house about the contest for Queen of the Fiesta, because one of Paula's nieces is a candidate. Paula's daughters are busy selling tickets for the contest, because each ticket sold is a vote for their cousin, and the girl who is elected queen is the darling of the colony. The Mexican-American radio and press are full of news of the coming fiesta. Plans are being made for the big parade downtown and the program of music and dances and speeches to be held in the civic auditorium afterward. Paula's mother and the other old people sit around the kitchen table and talk about *Cinco de Mayo* celebrations in the old days in Mexico— how beautiful the fireworks displays were, and how the bands played and the flags waved and the people danced in the plaza until morning. Nostalgia brings tears to the eyes of the old people who must celebrate the birthday of their homeland on foreign soil. During the fiestas patrias in San Jose, even Paula's sons, who have never seen Mexico, feel something of the patriotism which stirs the hearts of their parents and grandparents; and just as voices are raised in the cities and towns of Jalisco and Chihuahua, so they raise theirs to cry *"Viva Mexico!"* On such a day, they feel, it is a good thing to live in the colonia, where all men are their brothers.

Shops and Stores

The people of the colony want to buy many things which are not always available in Anglo stores. Their demands have led to the establishment of businesses aimed at the Mexican-American market. San Jose has dozens of Mexican restaurants, cantinas, and grocery stores which feature items of Mexican diet. There are also drug stores which sell the familiar Mexican herbs used in many homes.

Paula buys many of her groceries from a supermarket near her neighborhood because she feels that meat, produce, and canned goods are cheaper there than at the Mexican-American stores. There are some items, however, which Paula prefers to purchase from Mexican-American merchants. Tortillas of corn or wheat flour are best bought freshly made at a Mexican *tortillería* (tortilla factory); the sweet Mexican rolls which her husband likes with his breakfast chocolate she must purchase at a Mexican bakery; large sacks of pinto beans and the many sorts of chilies and herbs which flavor her cooking she buys at a Mexican grocery store. Paula's husband likes Mexican beer in the evening after work, and he often stops off at the neighborhood cantina to have a bottle of Carta Blanca with his friends and catch up on the neighborhood gossip. Paula's mother insists that her grandchildren be given herbal teas for various minor ailments, and then Paula must make a trip to a Mexican pharmacy for a jar of camomile or rue. Mexican phonograph records, magazines, newspapers, and pottery must be purchased in colony shops.

Because members of the colony want and purchase things which outsiders rarely buy, they are brought together in shops, stores, and markets. Even such a commonplace activity as doing the family shopping contributes to the feeling that Mexican-Americans in San Jose share a certain heritage and way of life with others of the colony, and are somehow set apart from outsiders.

Insulation of the Colony

It would perhaps paint a faulty picture of the San Jose Spanish-speaking colony to refer to its members as "segregated." It is true that many Mexican-Americans do live in communities and neighborhoods which are largely separate from Anglo populations, but Spanish-speaking families are scattered in many other neighborhoods as well. The type of spatial "segregation" which occurs in San Jose is less the result of discriminatory policies on the part of Anglos than of poverty. Many colony families must live in neighborhoods which they can afford. For these reasons, it is perhaps best to refer to the colony as "insulated" rather than "segregated."

Although Paula and her family have many contacts with Anglos, these contacts are either formal ones, as with teachers, doctors, or social workers, or very casual ones, as with store clerks. In the more intimate social contacts there is really no need for Paula to go outside the colony. Her relatives, compadres, and friends are Spanish-speaking people with whom she feels comfortable; there is no need to seek friends and associates among Anglos who have such strange ways and are so different from herself. And, too, Paula is not sure that they are kind and sympathetic. She has not suffered from open hostility or discrimination in San Jose, but she has heard many stories about such things in other parts of the state, and even in San Jose in past years. Paula's friends sometimes speak of Mexican-American men who were beaten by the police, of people who were refused service in cafes and restaurants, of Spanish-speaking boys who were arrested only for having long hair or wearing leather jackets. The people of the colony often say, "San Jose is not such a bad place for Mexican people—they don't give us much trouble here." But they remember that, in the 1940's in Los Angeles and Fresno and San Bernardino, gangs of Anglo soldiers and sailors and civilians broke into Mexican-American homes, wrecked furniture, beat boys and men, and even burned houses, while the police stood by and idly looked on [48]. The people of the colony do not suffer this sort of discrimination, but they remember it and fear that it may come back again. Their fear widens the gap between Anglo and Mexican-American and helps insulate the colony from the rest of the community.

In addition to the Mexican-American colony, several other ethnic communities have been established in the Santa Clara Valley. Sizable numbers of Portuguese, Italian, Japanese, and Filipino families have made their homes in the vicinity of San Jose. Yet these other immigrant groups exhibit little of the insularity and tenacity of tradition which characterize the Spanish-speaking colony. Valley people of Italian and Portuguese national origin have proved more inclined than Mexican-Americans to embrace the language, customs, and beliefs of their English-speaking neighbors.

An attorney of Italian background remarked that the present Mexican colony of San Jose is much like the local Italian community of forty years ago in which he grew up. His parents spoke only Italian at home, preserved Italian tradition, and made friends almost exclusively within their own ranks. Now, forty years later, descendants of Italian immigrants are virtually indistinguishable in speech, customs, and occupation from "old American" families in San Jose. The attorney related the assimilation of the Italian community to the fact that Italian immigration into Santa Clara County stopped almost completely about fifty years ago.

Mexican immigration, on the other hand, has not stopped. New people from Mexico come to live in San Jose every year, bringing with them fresh reminders of the language and traditions of the homeland. Even newcomers, such as the braceros who stay only a short while in the valley, contribute to the persistence of Mexican ways. Ancestral traditions are reinforced, too, by the proximity of California to the Mexican border. Many Spanish-speaking families each year travel to Mexico, visiting relatives and old friends and renewing old loyalties and beliefs.

It has been pointed out that insularity of Spanish-speaking groups is "both a cause and an effect of retarded assimilation. . . . Separate communities minimize the opportunities for cross-cultural contacts and thus delay the acquisition of Anglo cultural traits. Lack of Anglo traits makes for continued awareness of difference and a continuation of the tendency to live apart. And so the circle continues" [43]. Insularity is a great deterrent to the adoption of new medical ways.

Summary

The Spanish-speaking people of San Jose sometimes refer to themselves as the "colonia." The people differ in many ways, and find themselves divided by socioeconomic class differences, national loyalties, religious affiliation, provenience, and age differences. However, a sense of group loyalty within the colony is fostered by such factors as common language, common channels of communication, kinship, formal organizations, special events of common interest to Spanish-speaking people, Mexican-American business establishments, and a sense of separation from the Anglo population of San Jose. As a result of these influences, the social distance separating Paula and Armando from the Anglo community is even greater than that which separates them from other members of the colonia. They feel that they "belong" to the colony, and with its members they are comfortable and at home. They know what is expected of them and what they may expect in return. They find it much simpler to live within the colony than to deal with outsiders—strangers are full of surprises and unexpected behavior.

THE MAYFAIR COMMUNITY

Spanish-speaking families who live in the Mayfair District of San Jose are considered a distinct social unit by other Mexican-Americans of the region. The inhabitants of Mayfair are all members of the colony, but they are a little closer to each other than they are to Spanish-speaking people who live in other districts, sometimes miles away.

Because the people of Mayfair live in a single geographical area, they send their children to the same schools, worship in the same churches, and buy their groceries at the same stores. They also have in common similar standards of living and similar occupations.

Mayfair community shows the same tendencies toward social cohesion and cleavage which characterize the colony as a whole, but within the community similarities outnumber differences. For example, most of the people of Mayfair are medianos, working-class people who are neither well-to-do nor destitute. The men are unskilled or semiskilled laborers, with a sprinkling of skilled workers and foremen among them. Doctors, accountants, and proprietors rarely live in Mayfair. Nor is the population migratory; most of the people own their homes and have lived in the district for more than five years. As members of the same socioeconomic group living in a single community, they are a closer-knit society than the colony as a whole.

NEIGHBORHOODS OR BARRIOS

One of the chief characteristics of the Mayfair community is a tendency of its people to subdivide themselves into smaller neighborhood groups. Since Mayfair is a large community, its 3,000 Spanish-speaking residents cannot all know each other well. However, the district comprises about six subdivisions of smaller population, within which the inhabitants are in closer social contact. Each of the six neighborhoods, or barrios, as the people call them, contains from three hundred to six hundred Spanish-speaking persons living in an area of six to ten city blocks. Not all the neighborhoods are equally well defined, but in general the people of a single barrio know each other by sight if not always by name. Many families of a given barrio are related by blood or by marriage; some are immigrants from the same locality in either Mexico or the southwestern United States; some are fellow workers at the same factory, packing house, or fruit ranch.

A portrait of the way of life of the people who live in one of the Mayfair neighborhoods is presented in the following pages. True, all the barrios differ in some respects: some contain more English-speaking families than others; some have more substantial houses and more spacious grounds than others; the ratio of Protestants to Catholics varies from one to another; the residents have names for some barrios and no names for others. But most of the things that can be said about the customs and beliefs of the people of one Mayfair neighborhood apply as well to the rest of the community.

Brief descriptions of each barrio are presented here for the purpose of showing something of the range of variation which occurs in Mayfair. It is well to remember that although some houses are "substandard" and overcrowded, those in other parts of the community are very similar to houses in newly constructed "middle-class" housing tracts in many California communities. In one barrio, a family shrine decorated with religious mementos fills a corner of the living room; in the homes of other areas, the same corner may hold a high-fidelity record player or a spinet piano. The back yards of one barrio are piled with debris and the rusting skeletons of long-defunct automobiles; those of another neighborhood are expanses of well-kept lawn studded with rose trees.

Even within a single neighborhood there are sometimes marked differences in houses, yards, and the standard of living enjoyed by different families. The following sketches are no more than a general impression of the predominant features of each community.

Three of the six neighborhoods have names applied to them by the people who live there: Sal si Puedes, Sunset Barrio, and the Vollmer Tract. The others are unnamed perhaps because they are less well defined; we will call them San Antonio, Los Calles, and McCreery (see fig. 1).

Sal si Puedes

Sal si Puedes (Spanish for "Get out if you can") was the first neighborhood in Mayfair to be subdivided into house lots. It was once a settlement of Puerto Rican families who gave it its name because of the problems of navigating the streets which, before they were paved a few years ago, became mud holes during the winter rains. Later residents continued to use the name partly because of the mud but primarily with reference to the substandard housing and socioeconomic problems characterizing the community. The barrio is almost entirely populated by Spanish-speaking families, most of whom are Catholic. A Catholic mission church, the Chapel of our Lady of Guadalupe, is located there and serves as a focus for social activities in the neighborhood.

House lots are small, each having only a forty-foot frontage, as compared with lots fifty to sixty feet wide found in most other parts of Mayfair. Houses, too, tend to be smaller (three to five rooms) and less substantially built than those of other barrios. Although most homes have flowers and kitchen gardens, there are few lawns in Sal si Puedes. Parts of the area boast a number of large shade trees, however, planted by early residents in the 1910's. Streets are paved with asphalt, but there are no curbs, gutters, storm sewers, or sidewalks.

The barrio of Sal si Puedes will be described in more detail in later pages.

Sunset

The largest both in area and population of the six neighborhoods in Mayfair, Sunset barrio is about 80 to 85 per cent Mexican-American. It differs from Sal si Puedes only in having a less well-defined social

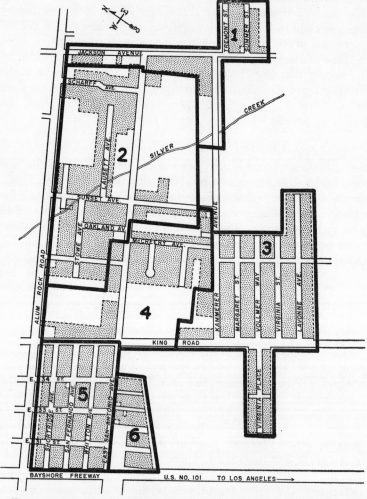

Figure 1. Mayfair barrios, 1955: 1. Sal si Puedes, 2. Sunset, 3. Vollmer Tract, 4. McCreery, 5. Los Calles, 6. San Antonio.

structure, somewhat larger and more substantial houses, and more yard space. Most of Mayfair's Spanish-speaking people live in these two neighborhoods.

Vollmer Tract

The Vollmer Tract is an area of new two- and three-bedroom homes, most of which were bought by World War II veterans. The neighborhood is adjacent to Mayfair Elementary School, which serves as a center for neighborhood activities. The area is about 40 per cent Spanish-speaking. Curbs, gutters, and sidewalks are found throughout the neighborhood, and the streets are well lighted at night. Most houses have front and back lawns, flowers, and small trees.

McCreery

The McCreery neighborhood occupies the geographical center of the Mayfair community, but has perhaps fewer Spanish-speaking families than any of the other five barrios. Only about one-third of its people are of Mexican descent, the other families being Anglo-American, Oriental, and Negro. McCreery can scarcely be thought of as a unified neighborhood; its residents have few social contacts with each other and participate little in community life. McCreery is the area that is "left over" after the other barrios of Mayfair are delimited. Houses and yards are slightly older than those of the Vollmer Tract, but are similar in size and state of repair.

Los Calles

Los Calles is the only one of the Mayfair neighborhoods lying within the San Jose city limits. Its streets are all lined with curbs, gutters, and sidewalks, improvements shared only with the Vollmer Tract. Many Anglo families live in Los Calles, only about 35 to 40 per cent of the residents being Mexican-American. Houses are generally five- or six-room frame or stucco bungalows built about twenty years ago.

San Antonio

The focal point for social activities in the barrio of San Antonio is a Mexican-American Protestant church, the Iglesia Apostólica (Apostolic Church of Faith in Jesus Christ), many of whose members live in the barrio. It is relatively small in size and population, and is perhaps more isolated from the rest of the community than any other of the Mayfair barrios. More than 90 per cent of its people are Spanish-speaking. Houses and yards are similar to those of Sal si Puedes, but there are fewer trees.

SCHOOLS

Five of the community's six barrios lie within Alum Rock Union School District, containing six county schools administered by the Santa Clara County Department of Education. Mayfair children attend four of those six schools: James Lick High School, Pala and Thomas P. Ryan Junior High Schools, and Mayfair Elementary School. The Los Calles neighborhood is within the San Jose city limits, and its children are enrolled in city schools.

Mayfair Elementary School alone lies within the boundaries of the community. All other schools which serve the area are in nearby districts of predominantly Anglo population. For this reason, Spanish-speaking children are in a majority at the Mayfair Elementary School, but make up only about 40 per cent of the enrollment of the two junior high schools and about 33 per cent of James Lick High School.

Mayfair Elementary School occupies a modern one-story structure built in 1950 to replace the old Jackson Avenue School, an ancient two-story wooden relic of the 1870's. The school population in 1955 was approximately eight hundred children, ranging in grades from kindergarten through the sixth grade. Approximately 65 per cent of the students came from Spanish-speaking homes. At the time of this study, the principal and almost all his staff were English-speaking Anglos.

Although a hot-lunch program is provided by the school, only 28 per cent of the entire enrollment take advantage of it [10]. Of those who do use the program, a disproportionate number are Anglo children; most Mexican-American students go home for their noon meal.

The school health service is administered by a school nurse who is employed half-time at Mayfair and a county public health physician who spends a half-day a week at the school dispensary. Children are skin tested for tuberculosis each year, and are immunized against smallpox, diphtheria, pertussis, and tetanus. Upon recommendation by the school nurse, children with chronic or recurrent health problems are given complete physical examinations by the school physician; parents are required to be present during these examinations.

A Parent-Teachers' Association and a Dad's Club have been organized at Mayfair Elementary School since 1950. Until recently, Mexican-American parents have taken little part in these activities. Before 1953, for example, only two Spanish-speaking mothers attended P.T.A. meetings regularly. In 1953, however, a Mexican-American woman was elected to an office in the P.T.A.; from that time on, other Spanish-speaking parents began to attend meetings. In 1955, Spanish-speaking parents made up about 40 per cent of the active membership and held three of the association's seven offices. In spite of an active effort on the part of school officials to draw Mexican-American people into school activities, many still feel that Mayfair Elementary School is controlled by Anglos: "The Anglos run the school to suit themselves—they don't care about us," one mother said. Although this attitude is widespread in the community, it is gradually being replaced by the new idea that "maybe they want us, after all."

Adult-education classes in citizenship and in beginning English are taught at the school two nights a week, and both attract a few Mexican-American residents each year. In the fall of 1955, thirty-one Spanish-speaking adults registered for classes; in previous years, as many as sixty attended evening school at Mayfair. Tomasa Cortez is a representative member of the American citizenship class. Tomasa is a widow sixty-one years of age who has lived in the United States since 1926. She lives with her daughter and son-in-law, who have partially supported her for several years. Tomasa works a few months each year at a cannery in San Jose, but she realizes that in a few years she will no longer be able to work and contribute her wages to the maintenance of the household. In 1954 Tomasa heard that a new Mexican-American group, the Community Service Organization, was helping some of the Mexican people to get their citizenship papers. If she were only a United States citizen, Tomasa thought, she could get an old-age pension when she was no longer able to work the long hours at the cannery. She persuaded one of her friends to go with her to a C.S.O. meeting at Mayfair Elementary School, and on the advice of that group, Tomasa enrolled in a citizenship class which was taught in Spanish. She attends the evening classes faithfully and in a few months will be eligible to take her citizenship examination. By the time Tomasa is sixty-six years old, she will have received her final papers and can then apply for an old-age pension.

Aside from church buildings, Mayfair Elementary School auditorium is the only large hall in the community available for public gatherings. Groups such as the C.S.O. hold regular meetings at the school. School officials have encouraged Mexican-American groups to use their facilities in the hope that members will develop a more active interest in school programs.

CHURCHES

Four churches in Mayfair hold services in Spanish and have chiefly Mexican-American congregations; of these, one is Catholic and three are Protestant.

Mayfair's Catholic church, the Chapel of Our Lady of Guadalupe, was built in 1952. Before 1952, services were held once a month in a small hall which, when the new chapel was completed, was converted into a youth center.

The Mexican-American Protestant churches in Mayfair are the Latin-American Assembly of God, Seventh-Day Adventist, and an independent Pentecostal sect, the Apostolic Church of Faith in Jesus Christ. All have Mexican-American ministers who conduct services in Spanish. There was a Mexican Baptist church in the barrio of Sal si Puedes, but in 1954 this church group moved into new quarters near downtown San Jose. Some members of that congregation live in Mayfair.

Churches are perhaps the single most important influence in formal community life. Many successful civic projects in the district, including public health programs, have been strengthened by church support, and without the endorsement of religious groups the effectiveness of such programs would be problematic. For a more complete discussion of the religious life of the community, see chapter 5.

STORES

Mayfair District is bordered on the north by Alum Rock Road, along which are found the principal business and commercial establishments of east San Jose. Alum Rock Road is an area of supermarkets, small groceries, used-car lots, furniture and hardware stores, filling stations, small cafes, and retail shops of all sorts. Several establishments in this district are operated by Mexican-Americans; the most highly patronized of these are grocery stores, Mexican bakeries, and a tortilla factory.

In response to Mexican-American demands, Anglo food markets in the area stock special items of Mexican diet which are seldom found in similar stores in other areas. Chain stores, for example, sell packaged fresh tortillas, canned *menudo* (Mexican tripe soup), *nopalitos* (leaves of the prickly pear cactus), and a variety of tomato and chili sauces.

In addition to the main shopping district along Alum Rock Road, there are five neighborhood groceries scattered throughout the residential area, three operated by Mexican-Americans and two by Anglos. Most families do the bulk of their shopping in the larger stores and make only incidental purchases at neighborhood markets. Small Mexican stores play an important part in neighborhood life as meeting places for the people. Women who drop into a neighborhood store to buy a can of vegetables or a box of cookies may stop to exchange greetings with a neighbor or gossip a few minutes with the wife of the storekeeper. Children gather at the store after school to drink bottles of soda pop or eat bags of peanuts. Older boys lounge around the store entrance or talk in low voices in huddles on a nearby corner. The neighborhood store is often the crossroads of the barrio.

THE ANGLO COMMUNITY

Most of the 1,500 non-Mexican residents of Mayfair live in the three barrios of McCreery, Los Calles, and the Vollmer Tract. Typically, they are working-class Anglos of north European ancestry; some are of Italian or Portuguese origin. Although a few families are long-time residents of California, many came during the 1940's from the south-central states (Texas, Oklahoma, Arkansas, Kansas, and Missouri) to work in war plants and shipyards.

A small community of Puerto Ricans dates back to about 1918. Although these Puerto Ricans are Spanish-speaking people, they generally hold themselves aloof from the Mexican-American community and are quick to remind outsiders that they were born on American soil.

Since 1950 a few Oriental and Negro families have bought homes in Mayfair. With few exceptions, neither group has had much social contact with their Anglo or Mexican-American neighbors. Their houses, incomes, and occupations are similar to those of Mayfair Anglos.

Since Anglo attitudes toward Mexican-Americans are so varied, they are difficult to describe simply. Some English-speaking people want to become better acquainted with their Spanish-speaking neighbors and welcome friendships with them. Others seldom invite Mexican-Americans into their homes, but do work toward closer relations between the two communities by participation in such interethnic organizations as the P.T.A. The majority of Anglos interviewed during this study, however, expressed an attitude toward Mexican-Americans which can best be described as "uneasy." On the whole, they know little about Mexican-American customs and values, speak no Spanish, and share with other California Anglos many of the popular misconceptions (for example, that Spanish-speakers are "transient," "lazy," and "always on relief"). They frequently have the notion that San Jose families "live just like they do in Mexico—they never change a bit, never learn American ways, and don't try to learn English." There is a tendency to base judgments of the Spanish-speaking community as a whole on the few obviously substandard areas in San Jose. Mexican-American families who live in well-built homes with lawns and gardens, those who deprive themselves of comforts to send their children through high school and sometimes through college, those who brave drenching rains on winter nights in order to study English at night school—these people, they believe, are "exceptions."

As a consequence of misunderstandings bred by social isolation, Spanish-speaking people in turn often feel "uneasy" with their Anglo neighbors. Many harbor a constant fear of open insult or discrimination—a fear based largely on past experience with a hostile and patronizing Anglo majority whose attitudes toward Spanish-speaking citizens have too long been governed more by fancy than by fact, more by ignorance than by knowledge.

Anglos have no monopoly on misconception and group prejudice. The Mexican-Americans of Mayfair view certain patterns of Anglo life with undisguised horror and others with amused tolerance. But as social barriers are scaled and commerce nurtured between peoples of different national origin in San Jose, disgust frequently gives way to sympathy, and sympathy is often replaced by understanding and appreciation of the traditions and values of other cultures.

The transition from group hostility to friendship is a new trend in the Mayfair District. Perhaps nowhere are the mechanics of this change more apparent than in the barrio of Sal si Puedes, where the transition from Mexican to American has so recently begun.

THE BARRIO

Although Armando and his neighbors belong to the larger San Jose colony and are residents of Mayfair community, they feel most at home within their own neighborhood, Sal si Puedes. Within the barrio the faces Armando sees are the familiar ones of family, friends, and neighbors; in his barrio more people smile and greet him as he passes, more doors open to him in hospitality, and more people stop him on the streets to ask about his health, his family, his work, and his plans for the future. In his own neighborhood, Armando feels, people really care about him. With the people of the barrio he works and plays and worships; together they watch their children grow up; with them he shares the pleasure and plenty of the good days; and from them he borrows strength and comfort in hard times.

Sal si Puedes differs from representative neighborhoods of the colony in three important ways: First, it is populated almost entirely by Spanish-speaking people; thus its residents are more isolated from Anglo customs and beliefs than most Mexican-American neighborhoods in San Jose. Second, partly as a result of social in-sulation, more Mexican patterns of life are retained in Sal si Puedes than in other barrios. Third, it is one of the poorer neighborhoods within the colony: most of its houses are small and overcrowded, back yards are often cluttered with shabby outbuildings and piles of rubbish, and many families must subsist on the precarious income from seasonal labor.

"Why are you so interested in that place?" a Mexican-American professional man asked; "The people are uneducated and poverty stricken—it's nothing but a slum, and most of our people are ashamed of it. You social scientists have a knack for seeking out the lowest-class Mexican neighborhood and reporting conditions you find there as typical of the whole Spanish-speaking community!"

There are two good reasons for basing this study on observations of life in Sal si Puedes. First of all, this study was designed to describe relations between Mexican-American people and Anglo public health personnel; but there are few public health problems to be studied among the "more representative" Spanish-speaking families —most clients of public health agencies live in substandard neighborhoods like Armando's barrio. Another reason for selecting Sal si Puedes is that in the daily lives of its people, Mexican customs and beliefs are evident and the effect of Mexican patterns in the treatment of illness is easily observed.

In spite of the fact that Sal si Puedes is an atypical neighborhood, much can be learned from its people about the Spanish-speaking community as a whole. For it is in similar areas that thousands of Mexican migrant workers have made their first real homes in California, after years spent wandering from place to place "following the crops." It is from such neighborhoods that their children, armed with an American education and knowledge of Anglo ways, have gone out to find better jobs, build better homes, and achieve a higher standard of living for themselves and their children.

PHYSICAL DESCRIPTION

Sal si Puedes is a community of seventy families living in small single-family dwellings which face four streets (see fig. 1). (There were only two multi-family dwellings in the barrio in 1955.) Houses have from one to six rooms, the average having 4.2 rooms and a bath. The average number of persons per dwelling is 6.28; living space per capita averages 0.67 rooms. (See figure 2 for distribution of sample.)

The house belonging to Armando Gutierrez is a typical Sal si Puedes home; Armando, his wife, and their four children live in a five-room frame house. The outside walls are clapboard and the roof is of asphalt tile. Armando and some of his relatives built the house themselves nine years ago on the front of a lot which he bought for $1,000. The lot already held a small three-room cabin which Armando and his family occupied while their new house was being built. The old house still stands on the back of the lot, and Armando's oldest daughter and her husband now live in it.

The Gutierrez house has a living room, a large combination kitchen and dining room, three bedrooms, bath, and a screened porch which is used for a laundry room.

The house lot is fenced on the street side with a wooden picket fence about three feet high. On the sides and back of the lot, there is chicken-wire fence stretched between cedar posts. In the back yard Armando's wife keeps a few chickens in a pen, and along the fences she has planted some rambler roses, dahlias, and a few parsley, peppermint, and onion plants. The only trees on the lot are a small elm in the front yard and a quince tree behind the house. The only animals kept by the family are the chickens and a dog.

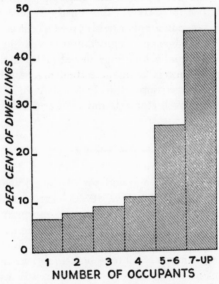

Figure 2. Household size, Sal si Puedes, 1955: number of occupants per single-unit dwelling (median: 6.28 persons per dwelling).

Armando's house is supplied with electricity, natural gas, and city water. Four-party telephone service is used. Until a few years ago, Armando used a cesspool for sewage, but after the cesspool was condemned by the district sanitarian, the house was connected to a sewer line.

Armando makes most home repairs himself; if there is a difficult job to be done, he asks his son-in-law to help him. During the rainy months of 1955, he built a front walk of wooden boards and laid gravel on the footpath between the main house and the rear cabin. He has recently laid new linoleum in the kitchen and bathroom and hopes to find time to repair his front fence and repaint the house soon.

The Gutierrez house is similar to most homes of the barrio; it is neither the best nor the worst dwelling of the area. Some homes are more substantially built and are less crowded. A family of four, neighbors of Armando, live in a six-room stucco house with a tile roof, concrete walks, hardwood floors, and plastered walls. Armando's compadres, on the other hand, with eight persons in the family, are crowded into a three-room cabin on the rear of a lot. (Figure 2 illustrates the range in number of occupants.) Several small houses in Sal si Puedes have been condemned and razed.

There are three public buildings in Sal si Puedes which are in use: the Catholic church, a small Catholic recreation hall, and a neighborhood grocery store, the Jackson Avenue Market. The market is small but well stocked, and is owned and operated by a Spanish-speaking family.

POPULATION OF THE BARRIO

In 1955, there were 422 people living in Sal si Puedes. Figure 3 shows the distribution by age and sex of the population as determined by a census taken in April, 1955.[5] There are several irregularities in the age-sex pyramid which require explanation. The larger number of males in the five–nine group than in the under-five group may be due to errors in stated ages of younger children. For example, one Sal si Puedes mother politely but firmly refused to answer census questions about her family. She apparently was not merely unwilling to have the field worker obtain the information, because she suggested that her sister, who also lives in the barrio, could provide the necessary facts. When her sister was contacted, she explained that, "The reason my sister didn't want to give you the answers to the census questions was because she was embarrassed to have to admit that she just doesn't remember exactly *when* her children were born." This leads to the conclusion that

[5] A complete individual census of the 400 residents of the barrio was intended, but the absence of many families during the spring growing season prevented the collection of data from all persons. Census materials were obtained from 281 persons (i.e., 67 per cent) of the area, and total figures calculated on the basis of this two-thirds sample. Data from 5 non-Mexican-American families residing in the neighborhood (3 Puerto Rican and 2 Negro families) were not included in the figures used in this study.

ages reported for some children might be off by a year or so, which could produce an irregularity in the age-distribution curve.

One of the most noticeable characteristics of the age-sex pyramid is the marked drop in the twenty-five–twenty-nine group, with a return to predicted numbers in the older age groups. This distribution bears out our observation that the barrio is composed of adults in the thirty–fifty age group and their dependent children and aged parents.

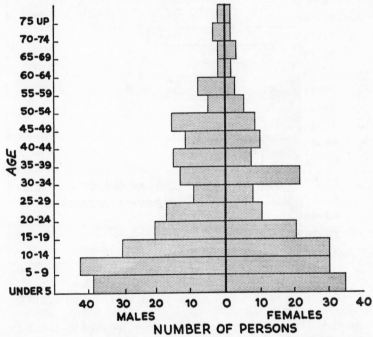

Figure 3. Distribution of population by age and sex, Sal si Puedes, April, 1955.

The married children of barrio families most often move out of Sal si Puedes to make their homes in other areas where housing is better. Most young adults in this age group are born and educated in the United States. With a better knowledge of English and with more education than their parents received they get better-paying jobs and move into more substantial residential areas. Young adults are also more likely to prefer Anglo patterns of living and Anglo associates than do their Mexican-born parents, who, even when they acquire enough money to move into better residential areas, often prefer to improve their old houses and live on in Sal si Puedes with relatives and old friends who speak their language and understand their ways.

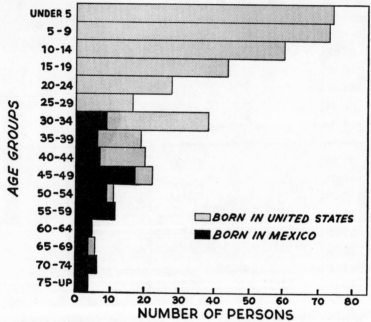

Figure 4. Place of birth by age groups, Sal si Puedes, April, 1955.

Another irregularity seen in the age-sex pyramid is the large number of females thirty–thirty-four years old. This increase can be explained in part by the fact that Sal si Puedes is a low-rent district and attracts a number of young mothers whose husbands, for one reason or another, are not in the home and cannot contribute to the support of the family. Some are widows, some are American-born wives of Mexican nationals who were illegally in the United States and who were later deported, some are separated or divorced, and a few are women whose husbands have deserted them and their children. These women often have no property, have several small children to support, and must find homes in low-rent areas like Sal si Puedes.

Place of Birth and Citizenship

The people of Sal si Puedes are 82.7 per cent American-born and 15.9 per cent Mexican-born. The remaining 1.4 per cent from other countries are largely natives of Puerto Rico. Most of those born in the United States are children and young adults, the older residents usually being of Mexican birth (see table 1).

TABLE 1

PLACE OF BIRTH OF SAL SI PUEDES RESIDENTS

Age	United States							Mexico			Other	Total all persons
	California	Texas	Arizona	New Mexico	Colorado	Utah	Total	North [a]	Central [b]	Total		
0–4	70	4					74					74
5–9	60	9	3				72					72
10–14	41	10	9				60					60
15–19	26	6	3		8		43					43
20–24	19	3	3		1	1	27				1	28
25–29	11	3					14					14
30–34	9	8	10	1			28	3	3	6		34
35–39	3	5	4				12	5	2	7	1	20
40–44	3	3	5	1			12	6		6		18
45–49		2	2	1			5	12	3	15	1	21
50–54			1				1	3	5	8	1	10
55–59								4	6	10		10
60–64								2	2	4		4
65–69	1						1	3		3	1	5
70–74								3	2	5		5
75+									3	3	1	4
Total	243	53	40	3	9	1	349	41	26	67	6	422

[a] North Mexico includes the states of Sonora, Chihuahua, Coahuila, Nuevo León, and Tamaulipas.
[b] Central Mexico refers to the states of the Central Plateau, principally Jalisco, Michoacán, Guanajuato, and Querétaro.

Most children nineteen years of age and younger were born in California; adults between the ages of twenty and thirty-five are in about equal proportion native Californians and native-born citizens from one of the southwestern states—Texas, Arizona, New Mexico, or Colorado; those from thirty-five to fifty-five are about two-thirds Mexican-born and one-third native Americans; the vast majority of persons fifty-five years of age and older are Mexican-born.

Aside from California, more people of Sal si Puedes were born in Texas than in any other state. Arizona was the birthplace of almost as many barrio members as Texas, and a few persons were born in Colorado, New Mexico, and Utah.

No person younger than twenty-nine years of age was born in Mexico. About 60 per cent of persons from Mexico came from the northern states of Sonora, Chihuahua, Coahuila, Nuevo León, and Tamaulipas. The other 40 per cent immigrated to the United States from central Mexico, principally Jalisco, Michoacán, Guanajuato, and Querétaro.

Citizenship tends to conform to place of birth, there being relatively few people of the barrio who have become naturalized citizens. Table 2 shows the proportions of American and Mexican citizens in the adult population of Sal si Puedes.

TABLE 2

CITIZENSHIP OF PERSONS 21 YEARS OF AGE AND OLDER IN SAL SI PUEDES

Age groups	Total	U. S. citizens		Mexican citizens	
		Number	Per cent	Number	Per cent
21–29	35	35	100	—	—
30–39	54	41	76	13	24
40–49	39	17	44	22	56
50–59	20	2	10	18	90
60+	17	1	5	16	95
Total	165	96	58	69	42

Although 42 per cent of the adult population of the barrio are of Mexican nationality, most Sal si Puedes families are long-time residents of the United States, a large majority having lived in this country for thirty years or more (fig. 5). No heads of families have lived in Mexico within the past five years, and only 10 per cent within the past twenty-five years. Their average length of residence in the United States is 33.6 years.

Mexican-American families migrated to California during two periods (fig. 5-B). Most of the long-time California residents entered the state directly from Mexico in the years following the Mexican Revolution, later coming to the Santa Clara Valley from southern California. During World War II large numbers of Mexican-Americans migrated from the southwestern United States to California to work in the fields and factories. The average length of residence of barrio families in the state of California is 22.4 years.

Some Sal si Puedes families have lived in the San Jose area for more than thirty years, but most of them arrived between 1940 and 1950 (fig. 5-C). On the average, barrio families have made their homes in San Jose for 12.0 years. On the average, however, a representative family has lived in the barrio only 8.4 years (fig. 5-D).

Summary

One of the purposes of this chapter is to point out that the people of Mayfair are, sociologically speaking, a relatively inaccessible

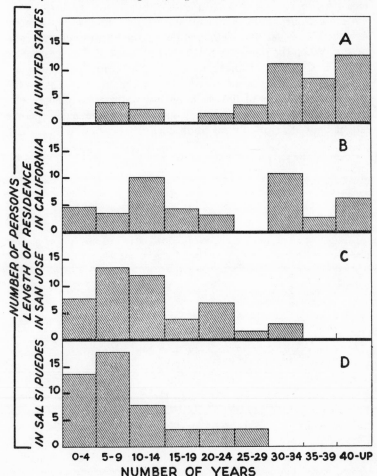

Figure 5. *Length of residence of heads of Mexican-American households, Sal si Puedes, 1955.*

group. They are members of an "insulated" enclave who feel a real sense of difference from both their Anglo neighbors and the "high-class" Mexican-Americans who are sometimes perceived by Anglos as colony leaders or spokesmen. Social distance poses persistent problems for health planners who hope to reach Spanish-speaking populations through influential local leadership. Some of these problems are discussed more fully in chapter 8.

A second purpose of this chapter is to give the reader a general view of the social and demographic characteristics of the community. When the people of Sal si Puedes speak of their position in the class structure of the community, they call themselves "los medianos"—the ones in the middle. The designation could as readily refer to other facets of life: in language, national allegiance, education, manners, and mores, they are "the middle ones," people caught between two cultural traditions.

3

LANGUAGE, LITERACY, AND EDUCATION

LANGUAGE, more than anything else, isolates the Mexican-Americans of San Jose from their fellow citizens. Most English-speaking people, long removed from the difficulties their own ancestors from Europe may have had with learning a new language in a new country, are generally unsympathetic with the failure of Mexican-Americans to speak English fluently. "There are some people who have been in the United States for thirty years who still can't answer a simple question in English," one Mayfair descendant of an "Old American" family complained. "Only a few of the educated Mexicans speak decent English—no wonder they can't make a living," another man remarked.

Certainly knowledge of English is not universal in Mayfair, but neither is it limited to "a few of the educated." Among Sal si Puedes families, there is a growing use of English in the home.

LANGUAGE

Sal si Puedes is composed of Spanish-speaking people: only four
persons of Mexican descent, two of them small children, do not
speak some Spanish at home. (See table 3.) Children from five to
nineteen years of age are generally bilingual: 62 per cent of them
speak both Spanish and English with relatives, 36.4 per cent speak
only Spanish, and 1.6 per cent speak only English. Although many
use only Spanish as a family language, all children in this school-age
group have some knowledge of English as a result of American
education. School children generally address their parents and other
adults in Spanish and talk among themselves in English.

The home language of about half of the people of the barrio who
are between twenty and forty years of age is Spanish, the other half
using both languages. Most of these adults who speak only Spanish
at home have some knowledge of English and some speak it fluently.

Of all persons in Sal si Puedes forty and over, more than three-
fourths speak only Spanish at home.

TABLE 3

LANGUAGE SPOKEN AT HOME IN THE SAL SI PUEDES BARRIO

Age group	Spanish only	English only	Both languages	Total
5–9	27	2	43	72
10–14	18	–	42	60
15–19	19	1	23	43
20–24	14	1	13	28
25–29	9	–	5	14
30–34	19	–	15	34
35–39	7	–	13	20
40–44	11	–	7	18
45–49	13	–	8	21
50–54	8	–	2	10
55–59	10	–	–	10
60–64	4	–	–	4
65–69	5	–	–	5
70–74	5	–	–	5
75+	3	–	–	4
Total	172	4	172	348
Per cent of total	49.4	1.2	49.4	100

Viewed as a whole, the population of Sal si Puedes is evenly divided in terms of home language: half speak only Spanish and half

are bilingual. Of those who speak only Spanish at home, some know enough English to be able to communicate fairly well in English; this brings the proportion of bilinguals in the neighborhood up to two-thirds of the total population, as compared with one-third who speak no English at all.

Bilingualism is a goal toward which the people are striving; most parents want their children to speak both English and Spanish well. "Some of the children who don't know any English when they start to school have a hard time here in Mayfair where the teachers don't understand Spanish at all," Teresa remarked. "In New Mexico where I grew up, it was different; in my home we spoke only Spanish and I had to learn English when I started to school, but it wasn't hard because my first-grade teacher was Mexican herself. She could speak to us in Spanish, and could use our own language to teach us English. Since my husband and I knew that our children would probably have teachers who don't know our language, we were always careful to speak some English around the house so that the children would have an easier time in school."

In theory at least, children are taught both English and Spanish during their preschool years. In actual practice most families use only Spanish in speaking to quite young children. When children reach the age of four or five, however, parents begin to address them occasionally in English in order to prepare them for school. Observation of one family, for example, showed that two preschool children differed considerably in their use of language. The older, four years of age, was addressed by his mother in a mixture of English and Spanish—in English most of the time, but in Spanish when she was scolding him or giving instructions. He answered her entirely in English, and spoke English to visitors in the home. The three-year-old child, on the other hand, spoke only Spanish, using occasional English words for material objects ("stove," "gun," "my bed"). The mother spoke to her younger child entirely in Spanish, and he replied in Spanish.

A few young parents in Sal si Puedes converse with their children only in English, although they may speak Spanish to one another. One young mother, when an Anglo visitor spoke to a small child of the family in Spanish, remarked with evident satisfaction, "You'll have to say it in English—she doesn't understand Spanish." When she was asked about language later, she asserted, "I don't care whether my children learn Spanish or not. I want them to learn good English and talk like any other American kids."

Although this attitude toward language is not unusual among younger parents, most people are not sympathetic with it. Doña Isabel reflected majority opinion when she asked, "Can you tell me why it is that young people don't teach their children our language? It's good for the children to learn English, because they must go to school here and learn to live with the Americans—but why must they give up their own tongue to learn another?"

Language means more to Mexican-Americans of San Jose than simply a way of conversing: the Spanish language is also a symbol to them of their existence as a community of people with a proud history and time-honored traditions and customs. Those who are either unable or unwilling to speak the mother tongue are seldom fully accepted as members of the community; they are likely to be thought disloyal to their own people. A teacher of Mexican descent was unsuccessful in organizing a youth group in Sal si Puedes because she was unable to gain neighborhood support for her program. A resident of the barrio attributed the teacher's failure to the fact that she spoke only English. "It's all right for an Anglo to speak bad Spanish—the people appreciate his trying to speak their language with them, no matter how poorly he speaks. But it's unpardonable for someone from a Mexican family to speak bad Spanish; people think that he's ashamed of being Mexican, and they don't trust him or his ideas."

Marta, a thirty-nine-year-old Texas-born woman, was fairly representative of San Jose Mexican-Americans in her language use. In her own home, she talked with Spanish-speaking relatives, friends, and neighbors in a colorful and colloquial Spanish, and was considered garrulous by her associates. With Anglos, Marta spoke English expressively although ungrammatically, but with them she rarely spoke of her feelings, emotions, or personal affairs. On several occasions, however, Marta was heard conversing in English when the subject shifted to her love for her children, her health problems, or her financial difficulties. Whenever the conversation shifted to a personal topic, Marta switched from English to Spanish without pause or hesitancy, and without seeming to realize that she had changed languages. When she was asked about it later, she explained that "there are some things we don't have the words for in English—like words for how we feel. For those things, it is better in Spanish."

For community leaders and Mexican-Americans in the public view (who generally receive more than their share of criticism from fellow colonists), proficiency in speaking Spanish is doubly important. For example, an officer in a San Jose Mexican-American women's organization was criticized by some members of the group "because she will never speak with us in Spanish."

Parents and grandparents are sometimes puzzled and hurt when older children and adolescents in the family refuse to speak Spanish, as they sometimes do. The mother of two teen-age boys complained, "I can't figure out what my sons are trying to do. I guess they just don't want to be Mexican. They won't speak Spanish even to older people who don't understand English—until their father gets mad and threatens to beat them. They could at least show a little respect for the old people!"

Many dialects of Spanish are spoken in San Jose. In addition to those brought in by immigrants from different parts of Mexico, there are several dialects that have been developed in the United States. An American-born college student told of some of the difficulties he encountered when he spent a year visiting relatives in Mexico: "Mexican-Americans have a hard time getting along in Mexico, because they are always set apart from other people by their dialect, among other things. In the United States it's pretty hard to keep using correct Spanish because you hear so much slang and peculiar terms. Even the Spanish radio programs here are full of slang and American expressions. The kids pick up a lot of *pachuco* talk, and some of their expressions get passed around among other people. Then there are Mexicans from other states of the United States who speak different dialects of Spanish, and the language gets all mixed up. It's easy to pick these things up, and before you know it, you're speaking an American dialect—not correct Spanish at all." (For a description of the pachuco argot, see Barker [2].)

A Texas-born woman complained that "there are a lot of Mexican people I can hardly understand, especially the educated ones from Mexico. When we first came to California, people here used to laugh at a lot of our expressions, and they used words that we didn't know. We don't speak real good Spanish—we admit it. We just talk to tell other people what we mean, not to use a lot of big words. We don't know many big words because most of us here haven't been to much school. We can understand our own language, but it's not good Spanish."

Some San Jose Mexican-American families are proud of the fact that they speak "correct" Spanish. "You must come with me to visit my mother-in-law," one woman said; "She is from an old Durango family, and I know you would enjoy hearing correct Spanish as a change from that terrible bracero dialect."

A characteristic of the language of many native-born Mexican-Americans is the use of English and Spanish words in the same sentence. Excerpts from a verbatim record of part of a young housewife's conversation with a friend illustrate the indiscriminate interposition of the two languages: "I don't think there's anybody nowadays like my husband—that's why quisiera que toda la gente fuera así, Vd. sabe, feliz como yo. . . . No, yo creo que both of them learned their lesson, porque dice ha que that's why she didn't want to wait for him to pay a divorce or anything, porque no le quiso nada—no quiere nada de él. And I guess that's right, porque ha sido otra, esperaba eso, don't you think so? . . . So, I don't think so. Maybe que later on, but I'm almost sure que no." [1]

Often, English words are Hispanicized, particularly terms for which there is no well-known Spanish equivalent. A typical remark heard in San Jose was, "Voy a parquear el troque en el driveway." ("I'm going to park the truck in the driveway.") Here the English verb "park" becomes "parquear," replacing the standard Spanish *estacionar*. Similarly, English "truck" is Hispanicized "troque," and substitutes for the standard Spanish *camión*. "Driveway," a word which is difficult to Hispanicize, is used without alteration in Spanish discourse.

A third trait of language among American-born residents of the Mayfair community is a tendency to substitute for little-used Spanish expressions literal translations from English. For example, at a jamaica or church "social" in Sal si Puedes barrio, the master of ceremonies, who mixed his Spanish and English rather casually,

[1] This quotation might be translated roughly: "I don't think there's anybody nowadays like my husband—that's why I wish everybody were like this—happy, like me. . . . No, I think that both of them learned their lesson, because she said that that's why she didn't want to wait for him to pay for a divorce or anything, because she didn't want anything of him—she wanted nothing from him. And I guess that's right, because if there had been something else she would have waited for that, don't you think so? . . . So, I don't think so. Maybe later on, but I'm almost sure that she won't."

was asked to announce the next item of entertainment, a Swiss square dance. Hearty laughter greeted his introduction of a *"Suizo cuadrado."* *Cuadrilla suiza* would have been an acceptable translation, but the announcer's imitation of English word order conjured in the minds of the audience the bizarre image of a "square Swiss."

The people of Mayfair are aware of the fact that English-speaking people sometimes dislike hearing them speak Spanish together. A patient at the Santa Clara County Hospital reported that "some of those *gabachas* [a derogatory slang expression for Anglo] act like they don't like Mexicans at all. A woman in my ward asked to be moved to another room because she said we jabbered in Spanish all the time and she couldn't stand it. But that's not true—we spoke both English and Spanish in that ward. But maybe now she knows how we feel sometimes, having to listen to nothing but English all the time."

Although there is pressure brought to bear on the Spanish-speaking people to speak English in the presence of Anglos, some members of the community accept the pressure without resentment. A Mexican-American boy, when asked what he thought of the rule at his school forbidding the speaking of Spanish on the school grounds, said: "I guess the rule is okay, because the other kids think you are talking about them in Spanish; it's just politeness." Adults are sometimes less tolerant of language pressures than children, however. "I don't see what all the fuss is about," an adult said in discussing the same school regulation; "Why should the teachers care, as long as the children speak English in class? If they're afraid the Mexican kids talk about them in Spanish on the playground, it's because the teachers are too lazy to learn a little Spanish themselves."

LITERACY

Although 98.8 per cent of the people of Sal si Puedes speak Spanish, only 45.6 per cent can read or write their native language. Among younger community members, whose education has been entirely in American schools (those from ten to thirty-five years of age), 70 per cent read no Spanish although it is the principal language spoken in their homes. Some young adults of Mayfair told of learning written Spanish for the first time as high school students, when they were taught it as a "foreign language."

For second generation Mexican-Americans in Mayfair, Spanish is a spoken language, learned by rote; they read it poorly if at all, and write only a phonetic approximation to correct spelling.

Table 4 shows that many people read English who do not habitually speak it. Thus, 49.4 per cent of the population speak only Spanish at home, but 76.5 per cent read English or both English and Spanish. Another 15.5 per cent are literate in Spanish but not in English, and 8.0 per cent of barrio residents over the age of ten are illiterate.

TABLE 4

LITERACY, SAL SI PUEDES BARRIO

Age group	Languages read				Total
	Spanish only	English only	Both languages	Neither language	
10–14	–	58	2	–	60
15–19	–	31	12	–	43
20–24	6	13	9	–	28
25–29	–	8	6	–	14
30–34	6	13	12	3	34
35–39	4	–	15	1	20
40–44	2	2	11	3	18
45–49	2	3	11	5	21
50–54	5	–	–	5	10
55–59	6	–	1	3	10
60–64	3	–	–	1	4
65–69	3	–	2	–	5
70–74	3	–	2	–	5
75+	3	–	–	1	4
Total	43	128	83	22	276
Percent of total	15.5	46.4	30.1	8.0	100

Those who claim to read and write neither language are all Mexican immigrants, most of them over forty years of age. Although illiteracy is characteristic of only 8.0 per cent of *all* barrio members, 16.8 per cent of all persons thirty and over are illiterate, and 32.9 per cent of the Mexican-born persons in the barrio are illiterate.[2]

Burma [8] pointed out that "Figures on illiteracy do not show the true problem" of Mexican-American education; "it centers chiefly in early dropping-out of scholastics rather than their failure ever to attend." During a health survey in the Mayfair community in 1944,

[2] The illiteracy rate listed is based on statements made by interviewed individuals themselves. It is possible that a few people may have claimed to be literate who actually were not. The percentage given, therefore, is a conservative estimate.

many Spanish-speaking people were reluctant to act as registrars and clerks because of difficulties with writing and spelling. A comparison of illiteracy rates of native-born and immigrant persons shows that American schools have had a pronounced effect on the people of Sal si Puedes, but there are still unsolved problems which prevent their receiving the full benefits of educational programs in their community.

EDUCATION

Just as the barrio of Sal si Puedes is composed of persons in lower-income groups, so the educational level of its people is markedly lower than either that of the Anglo population of the area or that of Spanish-speaking people in other San Jose neighborhoods. Table 5 provides a comparison between schooling of persons twenty-five years of age and over in Sal si Puedes in 1955 and three other 1950 population groups: California Anglos, California population of Spanish surname, and persons of Spanish surname in the San Jose municipal area.

TABLE 5

PERCENTAGE DISTRIBUTION BY SCHOOL YEARS COMPLETED: PERSONS 25 YEARS OF AGE AND OLDER IN FOUR CALIFORNIA POPULATIONS

School years completed	State of California [a]		San Jose, Spanish surname [b]	Sal si Puedes, Mexican-Americans [c]
	Anglo	Spanish surname		
None	1.3	10.7	8.8	35.2
Elementary				
1 to 4	4.3	18.6	21.0	23.0
5 to 6	5.3	14.2	15.6	14.3
7	4.4	6.3	5.9	4.4
8	16.2	13.7	15.9	14.3
High School				
1 to 3	18.0	15.4	12.4	7.7
4	27.6	12.8	11.7	1.1
College				
1 to 3	11.6	3.1	3.7	—
4 or more	8.5	1.8	1.0	—
Not reported	2.9	3.4	4.0	6.6
Total	100.0	100.0	100.0	100.0

[a] Figures taken from Saunders [43], p. 298. (Percentages calculated from data for 20 per cent sample of Spanish-surname population given in *Census of Population: 1950* [50].)

[b] Percentages calculated by the author from *Census of Population: 1950* [49]. (Based on a 20 per cent sample of 14 census tracts each containing 250 or more white persons with Spanish surname.)

[c] Percentages calculated from census of Sal si Puedes Barrio, conducted by the author, April, 1955. (Based on two-thirds sample of population.)

Figures taken from the 1950 United States Census of Population show that persons of Spanish surname in the state of California have generally completed fewer years of formal schooling than have

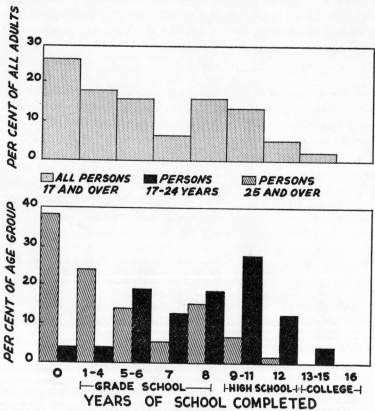

Figure 6. Educational levels of persons 17 years of age and older, Sal si Puedes, 1955.

Anglos; Spanish-speaking people within the City of San Jose, however, have much the same educational level as other California Mexican-Americans. The people of Sal si Puedes, on the other hand, lag far behind all three other groups in number of school years completed. For example, 58.2 per cent of persons twenty-five years of age and over in Sal si Puedes have completed fewer than five years of schooling; by contrast, the same educational level characterizes 5.6 per cent of California Anglos, 29.3 per cent of Californians of Spanish surname, and 29.8 per cent of persons of Spanish surname within the City of San Jose. Among California Anglos, 57.2 per cent have completed high school; percentages for persons of Spanish surname are 19.5 per cent in California, 17.4 per cent in San Jose, and only 1.1 per cent in Sal si Puedes.

These figures indicate that, although Spanish-speaking people throughout the state have educational problems, these problems are infinitely more pressing in neighborhoods like Sal si Puedes.

A comparison of educational levels of younger and older adult groups in the barrio clearly indicates that American schooling is making tremendous strides. Although persons seventeen years of age and over in Sal si Puedes have completed an average of only 4.8 school years (fig. 6-A), there is a striking contrast between educational levels of younger and older persons in this group (fig. 6-B). Persons twenty-five years of age and over have completed an average of 3.6 years of schooling, but those between seventeen and twenty-four years of age have completed 8.0 years. This great difference is due in large part to the fact that the older group contains all the immigrant population of the barrio, whereas all those under twenty-five years of age are second- or third-generation Mexican-Americans.

Although the younger adult group has on the average 4.4 more years of schooling than those over twenty-five, it seems unlikely that the children of the barrio who are now of school age will progress much further in their education than their brothers and sisters in the younger adult group. For example, in 1955 only 77.8 per cent of children of school age (six to nineteen years) were actually in attendance. The following table shows the differences in actual school attendance of children of three age groups:

Age	Total number	Number attending school	Per cent attending school
6–9	58	46	79.0
10–14	60	59	98.6
15–19	43	20	46.5
Total	161	125	77.8

These figures indicate that young children are sometimes enrolled in school a year or two later than Anglo children of their own age; thus, 21 per cent of the Sal si Puedes children six to nine years of age were not entered in the first grade at the expected time, according to California public school regulations. One child who was eight years and six months of age had not yet started kindergarten; he was a shy child, his mother said, and not ready to be away from home.

Although deferred enrollment accounts for some of the young school-age children not in attendance, it does not account for the fact that, in 1955, more than half of the youths fifteen to nineteen years of age had discontinued their schooling. Of these, some were high school girls who had dropped out around the age of seventeen or eighteen to marry or to accept jobs. Most, however, were boys sixteen to eighteen years old who had withdrawn as a rule in the eighth or ninth grade. The transition from junior high to high school is apparently a critical one for boys of the barrio. Many of them drop out at that time, but those who weather the first year or two of high school usually complete their secondary education.

It is abundantly clear that educational problems in the Mexican-American community are not confined to the immigrant population or even to the adult group as a whole; unresolved difficulties continue to plague Mexican-American school children living in Mayfair in 1955 and 1956.

The stories of Doña Isabel and her family illustrate some of these problems.

Doña Isabel is seventy-two years of age. She was born and reared in a small village in Zacatecas, Mexico, the fourth child of a poor farmer and his wife. There was no public school in her village in the late nineteenth century when she was a child and no opportunity for families of little means to educate their children. A rich man of the village, the *patrón*, who had large landholdings, sent his sons to a private school in a nearby town. A few village boys who were interested in church careers were given private instruction in reading, writing, and Latin by the local parish priest. Other villagers, among them Doña Isabel, remained illiterate. When she had been married a year, her husband moved his young wife north to the state of Coahuila, near the city of Torreón, where their six children were born.

One of her daughters, Paula, with whom Doña Isabel now lives in Sal si Puedes, attended school for three years in Mexico. When she was eleven years old, her parents decided to emigrate to the United States. They crossed the border at El Paso, Texas, traveling across New Mexico and Arizona into southern California. During the later years of Paula's childhood, her parents were migrant workers, moving about the state wherever there was work to be done. On one occasion, when Paula was thirteen, her parents lived for more than a year in a Los Angeles suburb. When classes began that year, Paula was sent to school to continue her education. This venture was short lived, however, because at that time she knew only a few words of English. Although she had completed the third grade in Mexico, she was put into the first grade in the Anglo school in Los Angeles until she had acquired a better command of English. Paula, at thirteen, was a large girl for her age, and she felt ashamed beyond endurance when she had to sit in a chair at one side of the room because she was too large for the desks designed for six- and seven-year-old children. A combination of language barrier, interrupted schooling which placed her far behind Anglo children of her own age, inadequacies of California schools of the 1920's to deal with non-English-speaking students, and casual parental attitude toward schooling conspired to terminate Paula's American education after two weeks.

A few years later Paula's family moved to San Jose, where she was married to a young Spanish-speaking man of similar educational background. In the 1930's the young couple moved to Sal si Puedes where their five children were born.

Paula's second son, Frank, is sixteen years old and a freshman at James Lick High School. He is two years older than most Anglo students in his class; he was a year late starting the first grade because the family was working that year on a prune ranch and did not return home until six weeks after the school term began. It was decided that Frank would wait and be enrolled in the first grade the following year. During his first year in school, Frank had difficulties with English. He found it very hard to learn both a new language and the things his teacher tried to teach him. He spoke English fairly well at the end of his first year in school, but had not learned his lessons well enough to be passed to the second grade. He spent another term in the first grade, and was nine years old when he entered the second.

Frank was discouraged by his failure to pass from the first to the second grade, but equally disheartening was his difficulty in understanding the things the teacher talked about and the things he read in his books. Things and people and stories that Anglo children had learned about before they started to school, Frank knew nothing about. It was a long time before he could figure out what a jack-o'-lantern was and what it had to do with the Feast of All Saints, *el Día de Todos Santos*. Although Frank had heard his parents and grandparents discuss many times the way in which the holiday was celebrated in Mexico, with all the people carrying food and paper decorations to the cemetery to adorn the graves, never once had anyone mentioned a pumpkin cut to resemble a face. He always felt a little at a loss when things that he did not understand were mentioned: how could he know about valentines or prairie schooners or Mother Goose or crossword puzzles? The American cultural tradition was so much a part of life for Frank's Anglo teacher and fellow students that they scarcely thought of it, but it was a vast store of knowledge which Frank had to learn slowly and by inference.

Gradually Frank discovered that he was getting further and further behind in his studies. Because his grades were poor, he was constantly afraid that he would have to repeat another grade and fall another year behind his age mates. But somehow he completed junior high school, and entered James Lick High. Many of his friends had become discouraged in school and dropped out. Some of them picked up odd jobs and always had a little money in their pockets and better clothes than Frank's parents could buy him. In high school, Frank discovered for the first time what it meant to be a Mexican-American boy in a school society dominated by Anglo students and teachers. Anglo students of his age often drove cars, wore good clothes, had spending money, and were usually a year or two ahead of him in school. Sometimes they made remarks in his presence about "dumb Mexicans." Now sixteen and in his first year of high school, Frank wants nothing so much as to quit school and go to work. He sees no future for him in school, does not want to wait until he is twenty years old to go to work and begin making money for himself, and is not convinced that graduating from high school will help him to get a better job. Frank has not dropped out of school before only because his parents will not let him; they keep reminding him that this is his only chance to get an education and prepare himself for something besides day labor. To Frank, at sixteen, the wages of even an unskilled laborer seem a veritable fortune, and continuance in school seems a painful and unrewarding chore. More and more he fails to attend classes, preferring to go to a movie or just loaf around the streets with some of his friends. Sometimes his father discovers that Frank has not been to school and becomes angry and threatens him with a beating. On these occasions Frank feels that even his own family is against him, and sometimes runs away from home for a day or two, spending the night with a friend in another part of town. It seems likely that this will be Frank's last year of formal schooling.

The mean school grade completed by Sal si Puedes residents is considerably below both the state mean and the average for the San Jose Spanish-speaking colony. Failure of barrio members to take fuller advantage of opportunities for formal schooling is a matter of concern to many people of the area. Educators, social workers, health personnel, and both Anglo and Mexican-American civic leaders are all interested in this problem. Teachers are becoming increasingly aware of the fact that Spanish-speaking children, especially those who, like the youngsters of Sal si Puedes, have had little contact with Anglos, pose special pedagogical problems. In the summer of 1955, a workshop for teachers was held at San Jose State College; the conference was devoted entirely to the problems of Spanish-speaking students.

Most people of the barrio concur that their children must have more years of schooling in order to get better jobs and enjoy a higher standard of living. A mother of several teenagers expressed her concern about education for her children: "My main worry is keeping the children in school, especially my fifteen-year-old son —he wants to quit and get a job. I've made him go on because I know you can't get a decent job without a high school education. My husband feels the same way I do—he only went through grade school; his family wanted to send him on to high school, but he wouldn't go. Now he is always saying that just because he isn't educated he's spent the best years of his life as a slave. That's why we want our kids to get an education."

Most parents, teachers, public officials, and civic leaders seem to agree that children from neighborhoods like Sal si Puedes need more education. But in spite of parental wishes, truancy laws, and teachers' workshops, in 1955 more than half of the barrio children over fourteen years of age had dropped out of school.

Some of the factors which make it difficult for Mexican-American students to continue their schooling are suggested by the above story of Frank's education. Three main aspects of Frank's life have contributed to his firm refusal to continue his education: the language barrier, economic problems, and minority-group status.

In reviewing Frank's educational history, it is clear that his troubles at school began with his imperfect understanding of English. Although he knew enough English when he entered the first grade to grasp much of what was said in the classroom, his English vocabulary was certainly much more restricted than that of his Anglo classmates. Most of what he had learned as a preschool child had been taught in Spanish, his home language; he lived in a predominantly Spanish-speaking neighborhood and had little need for an extensive knowledge of English. Frank's language problem was not that he spoke no English at all, but that he spoke so little English, and that little so poorly. In comparison with Anglo students his class performance was also below par, and he fell behind in his work and failed to be promoted at the end of his first school year.

Sal si Puedes children sometimes seem embarrassed about being behind Anglo children of the same age in school. One boy was heard to lie in order to hide the fact that he had spent two years in the first grade. Frank, like this boy, was a victim of an educational system much like that described by Burma [8]:

The normal procedure is to admit children at 6 or 7, carry on all the teaching in English, and trust that the child will learn the language and the content material simultaneously . . . most commonly the child learns both language and content imperfectly. The language handicap, difficult at any time, may become progressively worse until it becomes insurmountable and the child fails repeatedly and finally leaves school.

Although the language handicap—and the subsequent difficulty in adjusting to school—is responsible for part of Frank's scholastic problems, it is not the only reason that Frank, and others like him, wants to quit school. School-age Mexican-Americans are also affected by economic problems. Although Frank did not have to face the severe problems which his mother, Paula, encountered in her childhood as a member of a family of migrant workers, he was not untouched by the financial worries of his family. His first school problem arose from the fact that he was not enrolled in the first grade at the proper time: that year parents and children alike were working in the prune orchards in another part of the county when school opened. Many Sal si Puedes families are dependent on seasonal labor for their total annual income; money which is needed to support them through the winter months when no work is available must be earned during seven or eight months of the year. Sometimes the father, mother, and all the children must work during the harvest season to provide enough income. Often there is fruit to be picked during September and early October, and children may be four to six weeks late registering for school in the fall.

Some older children discontinue their schooling in order to go to work. Sometimes this decision is made with parental approval, sometimes not. Ramón was sixteen when he finished the eighth grade. He was the oldest of six children of a poor family. His father, a seasonal worker, wanted him to finish school, but Ramón thought that he was too old to be in school and also that he should be helping to support the family. He dropped out of school and started doing farm work. When Ramón's father died, he was left with the full responsibility of supporting the family. Unable to provide for his mother and younger siblings by farm labor, he decided to join the army so that his mother could receive a government allotment. Now married and with children of his own, Ramón insists that "all my kids are going to go to school!"

In addition to the fact that lower-income families need the wages that older children can earn, some Mexican-Americans leave school because they feel that they are not as well dressed as Anglo pupils and do not have enough money to spend. "I used to go to James Lick High," an eighteen-year-old Mayfair girl reported, "but I quit after the first year because I didn't have good enough clothes or enough spending money. Some of the kids there were stuck up and thought they were better than anyone else—they really used to make fun of me and the way I was dressed. You know how kids can be."

As members of a minority group, Mexican-American students face the additional problem of discriminatory attitudes in school. In part, these attitudes are the result of a difference in economic level, but mostly they arise from Anglo prejudice and discrimination.

The children of Sal si Puedes begin to be aware of minority-group status when they enter junior high school; they are only dimly aware of it in the earlier grades. One reason that discrimination goes undetected in elementary school is that Mexican-American students are not a minority. They constitute approximately 65 per cent of the enrollment of Mayfair Elementary School, approximately 40 per cent of the two junior high schools, and approximately 35 per cent of James Lick High School. For these children the transition from elementary school to the upper grades entails much more than a change of scene. For probably the first time in their lives they find themselves a numerical minority in a social group, and the attitudes of the English-speaking majority toward Mexican-Americans become increasingly significant to them. The effect of this transition on the children of the community is sometimes disturbing enough to result in withdrawal from school.

A juvenile probation officer in San Jose reported that most Mayfair boys referred to his office for repeated truancy want to quit school because of anti-Mexican prejudice. He expressed the opinion that many boys drop out because of poor counseling facilities, or no counseling at all. Almost all the Mexican-American students from Mayfair who were referred to juvenile authorities for counseling in 1955 remained in school; proper counseling facilities in the schools might prevent the premature withdrawal of many students.

An Anglo woman of Portuguese descent who attended both elementary and junior high school in a district of large Mexican-American population reported: "In grade school the American kids and Mexican kids got along fine—we all played together and there weren't any problems. But in junior high school it was a little different. The Mexican kids were poor and didn't wear very good clothes; they were clean, but most of them had a lot of brothers and sisters and their folks couldn't afford to buy them new clothes very often. The American kids in junior high got pretty snobbish about it, and used to make fun of the Mexican kids, especially the girls. The American girls used to give the Mexican girls a pretty bad time. The boys had a little easier time getting along, because they found out that if they acted tough and cocky that the American boys would respect them for that. Mexican girls got along with American boys all right, though. The American boys did try to embarrass them, though, and used to make pretty vulgar remarks to them."

"Discrimination" against Mexican-American students usually takes the form of teasing or verbal insults rather than open hostility or physical violence. Mexican-American students are sometimes poor, may have different customs, speak a different language, and are frequently behind in grade for their age; for any or all of these reasons, they may be teased and belittled by some of the Anglo students.

Failure to do well at school sometimes leads Mexican-American students to develop certain defensive patterns of behavior—cliquishness, formation of gangs, exaggeration of certain Mexican-American characteristics. A university graduate, now a San Jose businessman, reported: "I certainly had a hard time learning English when I first started to school; it was a fight all the time just to keep up with the average Anglo students. I would have to spend three hours sometimes studying what an Anglo student could get in thirty minutes. I was willing to put in the time, so I was one of the few that made it through school. It was very hard for Mexican students, and the teachers would run them down for being so dumb all the time. Most of them just got sick of it, and dropped out of school. But everybody wants to be admired for something, so a lot of the boys would form gangs and become pachucos, so that they could be looked up to for something . . . if they couldn't make it in school, they could at least make the headlines!"

One mother, whose teen-age son wanted to quit school after completing the eighth grade, said, "His father tells him to get his hair cut right [that is, shorter and without a "ducktail"], but he doesn't want to cut it off—he says he won't do it because his haircut is *chicano* (Mexican-American) style. I can't understand the boys—they don't want to stay in school because they say they can't dress and do things like the other boys, but they wear long haircuts and put pachuco marks [3] on their hands and that makes them look more Mexican and even more different from the other boys. I can't figure out what they want to be. Kids nowadays are hard to understand. They're just not raised like we were. When you try to get tough with them, they just run off or leave school. I used to be tough, but

[3] *"Pachuco marks"* are small tattoos, usually made with India ink and a straight pin, with which some Spanish-speaking adolescents mark the backs of their hands or fingers. The location on the hand varies, but the form of the insignia is nearly always a cross or some variation of the cruciform pattern.

I've decided you have to let them do a few things their own way and crack down on other things—let them have their chicano haircuts, but make them go to school!"

In spite of the problems of language difference, inability of parents to help children with difficulties in school work, economic pressures, and nonacceptance by some Anglo students, the educational level of Mexican-American children in Sal si Puedes continues to increase gradually. Educators and teachers show an increasing interest in the problems of Spanish-speaking children; counseling for students who are not succeeding in school shows promise of diminishing the rate of drop-outs. More and more children each year are born to younger parents who themselves have received some American education and are more aware of the importance of education and are better able to assist their children with school work. As more children are taught English and Anglo customs during their preschool years, more are succeeding in finishing high school and more are going on for vocational or college training.

4

MAKING A LIVING

THE PEOPLE of Sal si Puedes work hard to make a living. A few families have incomes which equal or surpass those of their Anglo neighbors, but many lack adequate food, clothing, and shelter. The high incidence of disease and the inadequate medical care which characterize many barrio families are the direct result of years of impoverishment. This chapter is directed to the following questions: How are high incidence of disease and inadequate medical care in Sal si Puedes related to low income? Do these families make any financial provision for unexpected illness? Do they have health insurance? To what extent are they dependent on public assistance? Are they trying to "better" themselves financially? Do they budget their incomes and spend wisely? If not, why don't they? Are they doing anything as a group to help their more needy members? What kinds of jobs do they have and do these jobs pay adequate wages? Are they trying to get better jobs?

Saunders [43] has pointed out that there is, "among Anglos of the Southwest, a great body of opinion and belief about the characteristics and abilities of the Spanish-speaking people." Among the supposed "natural traits" of Mexican-Americans are "laziness, as manifested in a disinclination to work" and "contentment with conditions as they are, as revealed in a lack of ambition and the absence of efforts to improve their status." The notion that the prime cause of poverty is indolence is shared not only by many Anglos but also by some San Jose Mexican-Americans who enjoy adequate incomes. A San Jose grocer of Mexican descent commented, "I don't know what's wrong with those people out there [in Sal si Puedes]—I think they're just lazy and don't care what happens to them."

The "lazy Mexican" theory is disproved by the fact that in the San Jose area Spanish-speaking people fill many jobs which require strenuous physical exertion. The economic problems of Sal si Puedes residents are acute; but they stem not from unwillingness to work but rather from poor job opportunities, low wages, and seasonal periods of unemployment.

TYPES OF EMPLOYMENT

With a single exception (the neighborhood storekeeper), the barrio residents are wage laborers, of which two-thirds depend on seasonal employment. A sample of forty employed male heads of families in Sal si Puedes showed the following percentages in various types of labor:

Types of labor	Per cent
Seasonal common labor (total, 65 per cent)	
Farm or orchard labor	25
Food industry labor (cannery, packing house)	20
Construction labor	20
Steady manual labor, nonagricultural	20
Steady semiskilled labor	15

Although 75 per cent of male heads of families are in nonagricultural industry, only 35 per cent of the total sample had secured steady employment; the remaining families were dependent on seasonal labor demands.

Although only 25 per cent of family heads questioned in 1955 were farm workers, the community is nevertheless largely dependent on agriculture. First of all, some men who reported that they were in industrial labor at the time of the survey (April) are commonly farm workers during summer and early fall when farm and orchard produce is harvested, and return to industrial day labor, such as road work or other types of construction, during other months. Agriculture plays a significant role, too, in the employment of women, children, and other dependents; even though the head of the household may be employed in industry, other family members often work in agriculture during the harvest season to supplement family income.

Agricultural labor is important, too, to people formerly employed in industry who can no longer get regular jobs because of advanced age or disability. Doña Isabel, for example, was employed for many years as a domestic worker. Now, at the age of eighty, she can no longer get regular employment, but each year she cuts apricots for drying during the harvest season. Dorotea, an eighteen-year-old girl who lives with her parents in Mayfair, said that she had to quit school to help support her family: "My father once had a good-paying job as a foreman in a mine, but the doctor made him quit because he kept getting sick with his chest. Later he tried to work for the Spreckels Sugar Company in Watsonville, but couldn't hold a regular job because of his health. So now he works in the crops— but farm work isn't steady and doesn't pay much, so I have to work to help the family."

The working people of Sal si Puedes have nearly all been farm laborers at one time or another. Most of them were migrant workers before they settled in San Jose. Some are still semimigratory, living in the barrio only during the winter months and moving each spring to fields and orchards in the valley wherever farm work is available.

There are several reasons for the agricultural background of barrio families: First, most wage earners or their parents immigrated to the United States from the central and northern plateaus of Mexico, where subsistence is almost entirely agricultural. Twenty or thirty years ago unskilled labor was the only kind of work available to most Mexican immigrants in the United States, and there have been few opportunities since for them to acquire the requisite skills and knowledge for more rewarding kinds of employment.[1]

[1] Saunders [43], in discussing economic problems of the Mexican-American people in the Southwest, says, "The economic position of the Mexican-American and Mexican rural population has not improved much in recent years . . . in places where the production of cotton, vegetables, and fruit is made possible by the periodic ap-

Within recent years, barrio workers have been moving from farm labor into nonagricultural jobs. In 1955, however, only limited types of nonagricultural work were open to Spanish-speaking people, except for the few who had a good command of English or special skills. Three categories of employment available to Mexican-Americans in San Jose were construction work, cannery labor, and fruit packing. All are seasonal industries with a peak labor demand during the summer or early fall and little or no demand during the winter. For a number of reasons family men in Sal si Puedes prefer to work in nonagricultural jobs if possible.

Julio, in the fall of 1955, got his first job as a road-construction worker; before that he had done only farm work. "I like construction pretty good," he reported. "It pays better, but isn't as steady as working in the crops. But, you know, a man gets older, and can't do farm labor so well—this summer I lost thirty pounds picking apricots and pears, but now I'm starting to gain weight again." Julio's belief that farm labor is more tiring than nonagricultural work—a belief not generally shared by other men of the neighborhood—is perhaps explainable on the grounds that he was being paid not an hourly wage but for the number of boxes of fruit he picked. Some of his friends commented, "Julio works too fast—he makes good money, but he works too hard." Alfonso, one of Julio's neighbors, said he preferred farm work to a factory job: "I got TB a few years ago, and I have to be outside where I can get plenty of sunshine and fresh air. I like it in the orchards pretty good, especially when the weather is nice." Alfonso, an experienced orchard worker, is employed by the hour, works for a single employer, and usually has employment ten or eleven months of the year. "I know how to prune trees and run the tractor, so I don't get laid off much. Most of the men aren't so lucky—they usually get only about eight months of work a year."

---

pearance of great numbers of migrant workers, wages have remained low and the level of living of the agricultural workers has shown little change. The poor working conditions and the low financial rewards received for their efforts have impeded the Spanish-speaking agricultural workers in acquiring the skills, knowledge, and attitudes that would enable them to function effectively in the Anglo cultural environment . . . in general it can be said that there are proportionately more persons in unskilled, low-paying jobs among them than is true of the Anglos. Lack of skills, poor educational background, unfamiliarity with Anglo ways, and, at times, discrimination by Anglos, all operate to keep many . . . Spanish-speaking persons at the bottom of the economic ladder."

Agricultural workers have more acute financial problems during periods of unemployment than do nonagricultural laborers. "The present Social Security Act is of less than normal benefit to them, for agricultural workers are specifically excluded from Old Age and Survivors Insurance, Unemployment Insurance, and Industrial Accident Insurance" [8]. A cannery worker, packing-house employee, or construction laborer is, during seasonal layoffs, eligible for unemployment compensation. Vincente, a cement-construction worker, reported that "one year, 1953, I was only off work two weeks. I guess God was taking care of me, because most years there just aren't any jobs in the rainy season [November through February]. You might make about two days—thirty-five dollars a week, but if you go on unemployment compensation you get thirty-three dollars a week. For two bucks a week more, why should you work in the wet and cold?" [2] Julio, who first became a construction worker in 1955, expected to continue working during the winter, even if he earned only $35 a week for two days' labor. Most other men who are eligible prefer to draw unemployment compensation for not working at all; Julio, however, is not yet a citizen of the United States, and would receive no unemployment benefits.

Wages in agricultural labor are considerably lower than in either agricultural or nonagricultural industries. Average wages for men in farm labor in Santa Clara Valley in 1955 were between 90 cents and $1.00 an hour. Average hourly wages for piecework, in which most women and older children were employed, were considerably lower, sometimes as little as 30 cents an hour.

In contrast with agricultural wages, cannery wages in 1955 were $1.39 an hour for women and $1.55 to $2.16 an hour for men. Foremen earned as much as $2.50 an hour. Fruit-packing wages were in the same range, women receiving $1.39 an hour and men $1.55. Packing-house forewomen earned $1.54 and foremen $2.07 an hour. Of the principal industries in which Sal si Puedes people were employed, construction labor was the most highly paid: unskilled workers in 1955 received $2.17 to $2.50 an hour.

The higher wages received by nonagricultural workers are due in

[2] Burma [8] has remarked that "Mexicans frequently have the reputation of liking relief. This is at least partially true, but it stems from the pitifully low wages they receive when working, rather than any special laziness or lack of moral fiber, as has been frequently charged. A man whose children are better fed and clothed by social welfare than they are when he is fully employed may be foolish to work."

part to the unionization of industry in the San Jose area. Farm workers, on the other hand, have no union representation and no collective-bargaining power. There have been attempts for the past several years to organize unions among farm workers in the Santa Clara Valley as well as in other parts of the state. One Sal si Puedes agricultural laborer remarked that attempts to unionize farm workers had so far been unsuccessful, in his opinion, because the men are not seriously interested in farm labor. "Our people here in northern California are trying to get off the farms and into other kinds of work where they won't get laid off so much. They fall back on the crops when there isn't anything else to do. I think that since there is such a drive on the part of the people to get into industry, they aren't really interested in the conditions of agricultural employment. All these things make it hard for the unions."

Many people in San Jose, both Anglos and Mexican-Americans, are convinced that unionization is the only practical means for providing steady employment, better working conditions, and a living wage for agricultural laborers. A San Jose Mexican-American leader, in discussing attempts by the C.I.O. to organize farm workers in the Imperial Valley, said he thought this sort of work was among the most important jobs to be done at this time for the Spanish-speaking people: "If general improvement in standard of living among our people is to come, it will have to come through reform in agricultural labor. Emphasizing industrial problems is foolish, since Santa Clara County is an agricultural area and will probably continue to be so for years. There isn't really enough industrial development here to furnish jobs for the Mexican people—and they will have to depend on farm work for at least another ten years. You can't help the Mexican people right now by assuming that they will all go into industry and ignoring the problems of the migratory workers."

An Anglo professional man who favors unionization of farm workers had similar comments: "In October, 1954, there was about a 30 per cent unemployment rate among Spanish-speaking wage earners in the county—this figure refers just to those who are permanent residents of California. This situation isn't due to lack of labor demand, but to the import of Mexican nationals by local farmers and ranchers. Farmers prefer Mexican nationals to local residents because the braceros will work for fifty cents an hour plus some sort of sub-standard housing, whereas local laborers demand from seventy-five cents an hour up, and demand better housing facilities if housing is to be furnished in lieu of part of their wages. Ranchers and farmers also know that nationals will work longer hours and work overtime at straight wages, if requested. Resident workers, on the other hand, ask for overtime pay at an increased rate.

"One prune grower in the Santa Clara Valley is now building three hundred housing units in preparation for next year's growing season, and is planning to import three hundred families of Mexican nationals to pick his prune crop. This same rancher utilized local labor last year. If this trend keeps up, it can easily lead to further impoverishment of local Mexican-American families. I'm certain that an agricultural workers' union is the only solution to this problem now."

Braceros are an unpopular group among Spanish-speaking residents of San Jose. The people fear the increasing tendency on the part of valley growers to contract for imported Mexican labor. In August, 1954, there were 4,500 braceros employed in Santa Clara County, constituting 16 per cent of the total number of hired farm workers. A year later, in August, 1955, the number had increased to 9,883, or 23.5 per cent, of all agricultural workers hired in the county. California State Farm Labor *Reports*, Santa Clara County Data Sheets for August 7, 1954, and August 6, 1955, show the following numbers of agricultural laborers in various categories, excluding farmers and unpaid family members:

Farm workers	1954	1955
Total hired in Santa Clara County	28,150	43,920
Hired year around	6,250	7,900
Hired temporarily		
Local	10,400	14,800
Nonlocal	7,000	11,900
Out-of-state	2,500	2,017
Mexican Nationals	4,500	9,883

The general feeling among resident Mexican-Americans is that the importation of Mexican nationals increases job competition and keeps farm wages pitifully low.

Julio reflected the opinion of most Sal si Puedes residents about Mexican nationals: "I've been following the crops in California for about twelve years, and I still don't know if I'm for or against the braceros. I guess that's because I first came to this country as a bracero myself in 1941, and know something about their problems. But I also know that when the braceros come in, the wages stay very low; that's pretty bad for people who have to earn their whole year's income just during the harvest season. I don't know how much of the money the braceros earn ever gets back to Mexico, either, because so many of them are single men with no families. Or they are men who are not very good husbands or fathers—they come to the United States to get away from their responsibilities to their families in Mexico. When I was a bracero myself, I knew both kinds of men, and I know they spend their wages here in the United States having a good time and never get back to Mexico with much money. If all the braceros were like that, I would be against them, but I know some really want to work and need the money. Take me, for instance: I was poor in Mexico and would never have made a decent living if I hadn't got the chance to work as a bracero. I came in as a contract worker for two years and made enough contacts so that the next year I could immigrate to the United States.

"Most of the ranchers around here like the braceros—they have to work on a contract and can't leave until the work is done or they won't get paid. They can't try to get higher wages by striking, and they'll work for less money. That way a rancher can count on having steady workers for his crop. All these things make it hard for me to say if braceros are a good thing or a bad thing."

Since almost two-thirds of Sal si Puedes family heads are employed in seasonal work, there are winter months when purses are lean and pantries are unfilled. In order to ease the economic distress occasioned by seasonal unemployment, many women and children work long hours during the harvest season. A common pattern of seasonal variation in employment is illustrated by the following family: The husband is an unskilled construction worker seasonally employed. The family is largely dependent on his wages, but family income is supplemented by other members. The wife, Consuelo, earned $25.00 in January, 1955, by sewing for the children of a neighboring family. This money was sorely needed during the winter when the husband was unable to find work. From May to July, Consuelo was able to earn additional money by taking in two boarders, Mexican nationals in San Jose for the summer harvest. In August, when Consuelo's boarders left San Jose, she got a job at a cannery for the entire month. The oldest son of this family was able to find work seven months in 1955, three months in construction and four in agriculture. The younger children worked in the fields and orchards from June to September. All members of the family were unemployed during November and December, their sole income in these months coming from the husband's unemployment compensation of thirty-three dollars a week.

For Consuelo's family and their neighbors, the seasonal cycle of labor and leisure divides the year into two main parts. During the warm months of the year almost everyone works—men, women, and children; but when the crops are harvested, the orchards of the valley stripped of fruit, the canneries and the packing houses closed for the season, and the first winter rains begin to fall, then only a few have jobs in factories and stores.

For most families, summer days begin long before the sun is up. By the time the gamecocks in Don Rafael's back yard begin to crow, the barrio is already rousing itself. Consuelo is one of the first to begin her day's work, rising at four o'clock to make the day's supply of tortillas for her family and the migrant boarders for whom she cooks. "It's a hard life for a woman who has no daughters to help with the cooking," she often complains to her friends. Consuelo's neighbor, Rosa, gets up an hour later to prepare breakfast for her family. Rosa's husband, Ismael, leaves the house at six o'clock to drive the fifteen miles to the apricot orchard where he is a foreman. At about half-past six Rosa and her ten-year-old daughter hear a car stop at the front gate and hurry outside to ride in a neighbor's car to a farm four miles away where they will pick strawberries. As they leave the house, they meet several women who are just coming home from their jobs on the night shift at canneries or frozen-food plants. These women go home to prepare breakfast and lunches for their husbands and sons and get them off to work, eat strangely timed early morning suppers, hastily straighten their houses, and go to bed.

By eight o'clock the sounds of voices and car engines have died away and once more the neighborhood streets are empty and still. Summer days in the barrio are hot and dusty, and the silence is broken only by the barking of a dog down the street or the voices of two or three small children who have been left behind in the care of an aged grandmother or an older sister.

When jobs are available during the summer months, everyone

who is physically able is expected to work. Elvira, a young mother whose fourth child was born early in the summer of 1955, complained that she was "missing the season" because she had to stay at home with her new baby. She felt that she had a good reason for remaining unemployed during the summer, but remarked that her cousin, Mary, had no excuse for not working: "She got a job in the cannery yesterday, but she only worked four hours and then had to quit. She said she was sick, but I think she is just lazy."

During the summer months, most people finish their day's work between five and six o'clock. The trip from the fields and orchards back to town may take almost an hour, and farm workers reach Mayfair about half-past six or seven o'clock in the evening. After that time, there is food to be bought for the evening meal and the next day's breakfast and lunch. The people reach home with their grocery purchases, bathe and change into clean clothes, prepare and eat supper, and go to bed between nine and ten o'clock.

When the rains begin to fall in November of each year, the barrio takes on a different character. The winter season is the time of year when people send their children to school, fulfill social and religious obligations, repair their houses, attend parties, and visit with friends. From November to March, although times are hard and there is little money to spend, people have leisure time in which to enjoy the social life of the neighborhood. In November and December, a festive air fills the homes of Sal si Puedes. The people usually have new clothes, bought with money earned during the harvest season. The women are busy with preparations for the church bazaar, Thanksgiving and Christmas holidays, or plans for parties, baby showers, and birthday celebrations. Men work around the house or on the automobile. Some of the people take winter vacations to visit relatives in other parts of California or in other states. For the people of the barrio, just as summer is the time for work, winter is the time for play, for gossip, for visiting, and for "living life."

OCCUPATIONAL GOALS

Sal si Puedes workers would like to have better jobs and earn more money. Julio spoke for many of his neighbors when he said, "I think a lot of Americans have a strange idea about how the Mexican people like to live. They imagine that we like to live in shacks and eat only beans and tortillas, because that's what we're used to. This is not true—even in Mexico the poorest man knows about meat, eggs, fruits, vegetables, and milk. It is the same way with us here—we would rather live in a house with a good floor and a tight roof than in a shack; we like to eat meat when we can buy it. But sometimes we can't."

The immediate occupational goal of most men of the barrio is to get a "steady job" without seasonal layoffs. A nonseasonal job is considered something of a prize even though hourly wages may be lower than the current rate for construction or general labor. Men who have year-round jobs often are on the lookout for openings at their place of employment, and pass the news of an opening on to relatives or compadres. For example, Pete, a machine operator at a manufacturing plant, commented that his employer was looking for several new men: "I sure would like to get my compadre Chavez a job there—he's not working right now. Six years ago I finally got my cousin working at the plant as a janitor, but it took me a solid year to get him in. They didn't want to hire him because he couldn't read or write, but his wife helped him and he studied enough so that he could read the orders. He's been working there ever since. I don't know about my compadre, though, because he can't read, either."

Although most wage earners are unskilled workers, a few are beginning to learn trades and crafts. Some had the opportunity during military service or after the war, through the G. I. training program, to learn vocational skills. Pío, a World War II veteran, was a manual laborer before the war. After his discharge from the armed services, the Veterans Administration helped him to get an apprenticeship to learn shoe repairing. In 1955, Pío had completed his apprenticeship and was looking for a location in east San José to open his own shop. Ramón, a barber, became an agricultural worker when he was eighteen years old: "When I was nineteen or twenty, I was drafted into the army. When I got out, I thought I might like to go back to school, but I was too old for that. So I got some G. I. money and went to barber college instead. Now I ought to save some money from my job and buy some houses to rent so I'll have some money when I get old."

A number of people were asked what sort of work they would like to do; these were some of the replies: "The Mexican fellows here like to be a mechanic or work in a gas station. Some like to be a barber or do shoe repairing." "What I'd really like to do is start a restaurant in east San Jose—a nice clean place where you could get really good Mexican food. A cafe and bar on a good corner would be nice—you could really get ahead that way." "My job is okay for right now, but some day I'd like to get hold of some houses to rent." "I'd like to go into the shoe-repair business for myself. I've got the machinery, but I need a location and some money for supplies to set up in business." "Ismael [the speaker's husband] really likes orchard work. He likes to work outdoors and get plenty of sunshine. When we can save some money, he thinks he wants to buy a little place of his own and put in fruit trees." "My brother is seventeen now and he wants to finish school so he can be an airplane mechanic. He asked my mother if he could finish school and she said okay, if that's what he really wanted to do."

Sal si Puedes men, as the above comments indicated, want to get into types of work in which they are self-employed. Trades such as barbering, shoe repairing, and garage work are particularly attractive because men in these trades can, with a little capital, open their own places of business. Many would like to become enterpreneurs or small proprietors. None mentioned professional or clerical work as an occupational goal, perhaps because of the educational level required for these positions. Many parents, however, hope that their sons will have the opportunity to become professional men. "Joe's father wants him to be a lawyer," one mother said; "he doesn't want Joe to have to work hard all his life like he's had to do and have nothing to show for it when he gets old." "My son is twenty years old now and for all his life I've been waiting for the day when he would be an engineer. Now he's going to graduate from college pretty soon—that's gonna be the best day of my life!"

The most desirable career for women is thought to be that of wife and mother. Few women want jobs themselves. They want their husbands to have steady employment at good wages and their children to receive enough education to enable them to work at something other than day labor. Some of the teen-age girls in the barrio, however, would like to work for a few years before they are married: "I don't want to get married right away," one eighteen-year-old girl asserted; "My mother was almost thirty when she got married, and I think that's soon enough. If you get married when

you are real young, you begin to have a family before you can afford
to raise them. I'd rather be a salesgirl for a while first. I'd like to
buy some clothes and a car—then get married later. Right now
I've got other fish to fry!" "I've always wanted to go into nursing, ever
since I could talk," another unmarried girl reported. "I know I won't
make much money, but I'll get a lot of satisfaction out of it." Nursing
is an attractive occupation also for some young married women of
the barrio. One woman who worked as a nurse's aide for part of
1955 said, "You know, the thing I wish for most is that I could say
I was a registered nurse. That's something I've always wanted to
be—especially psychiatric nursing, because my mother has that kind
of disease, and I'd like to know more about how to help her."

Sal si Puedes residents like to talk about "good jobs" and "being
your own boss," but many of them realize, like Paula, that "my
husband and the other men have big ideas, but I'm afraid nothing
will ever come of them—maybe for our children, yes, but not for
us in our lives." The dream is a shop or a store or a farm of one's
own; the reality is quite different. "Steady jobs" are hard to find
unless a member of a man's extended family group is regularly
employed and can "get him in." Available jobs for Spanish-speaking
people are still mainly physically demanding, poorly paid, and seasonal; many families survive the long winter months of unemployment only through the summer labor of wives, children, and even
aged dependents. When the summer's wages are depleted, survival
depends on the charity of friends and relatives and on public assistance. But even in the face of poverty the dream of "something
better" dies hard; it touches the lives of almost everyone in the
barrio, even those who are very young. One rainy day in 1955,
toward the last of November, Marta was entertaining a visitor. The
talk was of the coming Christmas holidays and Marta's worry about
money to buy presents for the children. Four-year-old Ricky piped
up to assure his mother that he already had her Christmas present
selected: "I'm gonna buy you a refrigerator for Christmas," he announced. When his mother asked how he was going to get the
money, he said "I'll pick it up off the ground." Marta laughed and
explained that Ricky thought prunes and money were the same
thing. Ricky laughed too, and added, "Sure, I'll pick enough prunes
to get a refrigerator," and (to the visitor) "I'll be so rich that I
might buy you one, too!"

FAMILY INCOME

Annual earnings of Sal si Puedes families vary with the number of members who work and with the kinds of jobs they have. In 1955, representative families of average size (six or seven members) in which the principal source of income was the husband's wages had the following estimated [3] annual incomes:

Employment of principal wage earner	Estimated annual family income	
	Range	Average
Seasonal farm labor	$1,500–4,000	$2,800
Seasonal nonfarm labor	1,800–5,000	3,600
Steady manual labor	3,000–5,500	4,500
Steady semiskilled labor	4,000–6,000	5,000

The above estimates include wages of the family head and supplementary income from summer earnings of other family members. Annual income was often considerably greater for families with several adult children who were employed full or part time than it was for families with only one working member.

Because there is so much variation in size and composition of households, figures on average family income fail to provide an adequate index of living standard. Perhaps more significant are estimates of per capita income. Table 6 shows estimates of family and per capita incomes for eight households during the year 1955. Judging from family income alone, it would seem that Family 3 with an annual income of $2,970 should be in a poorer financial situation than Family 6, whose yearly earnings totaled $11,895. Yet the two families live in similar houses, wear similar clothes, and eat similar food. The observed similarities in standard of living of the two families are dependent not on total family earnings, but on comparable per capita incomes. The fifty-seven persons in the eight families described had an annual mean per capita income of $752

[3] People of the barrio were not always willing or able to give exact figures on annual family income. A number of families were asked to estimate their yearly earnings and, wherever possible, these figures were checked through social service records of various county agencies (records of district nurse, social service department of county hospital). In addition, for higher-income families whose earnings were not recorded by county agencies, a San Jose tax accountant furnished estimates from his files of gross family income reported on tax returns. For obvious reasons, the tax accountant withheld the identities of his clients, except for the type of employment of the principal wage earner.

and a median per capita income of $780 in 1955. These figures are not to be taken as the barrio average, however, since the sample of families described is small and is not a representative one. There are a number of neighborhood families whose support is completely dependent on public assistance of some sort—widowed or deserted

TABLE 6

ANNUAL EARNINGS AND FAMILY INCOME OF EIGHT SAL SI PUEDES FAMILIES

Family number	Wage earners	Source of income	Individual annual wages	Annual family income	Family members	Annual per capita income
1.	Husband Wife & six children	Factory Agriculture	$3,745 575	$4,320	8	$ 540
2.	Husband Wife Son	Construction, cannery Domestic, cannery Construction, agriculture	2,550 270 1,180			
	Three sons	Agriculture Unemployment comp.	550 350	4,900	6	816
3.	Husband Wife & daughter	Agriculture Agriculture, cannery	2,500 470	2,970	3	990
4.	Husband Wife Son	Common labor Domestic Agriculture	2,500 640 40	3,180	6	530
5.	Husband Wife Husband's mother	Construction Home nursing Agriculture	4,960 25 95	5,080	4	1,270
6.	Husband Son Son Son Daughter-in-law Wife & four children	Agriculture Agriculture Construction Factory Cannery Agriculture Unemployment comp.	1,850 2,100 2,700 3,200 820 900 315	11,895	13	915
7.	Husband	Machine shop	4,680	4,680	6	780
8.	Husband Wife Son Daughter-in-law Daughter Two sons	Factory Cannery Agriculture Cannery Cannery Agriculture	2,860 750 1,440 380 380 45	5,855	11	532

mothers and their children dependent on state aid, old people on pensions or supported by the meager contributions of relatives, and the families of sick and disabled persons who must depend on county relief for survival.

Table 6 shows that the heads of the eight families described contributed an average of 60 per cent of all money received during the year, other family members contributed 38.7 per cent, and 1.3 per cent was received from government agencies in the form of unemployment compensation. In Family 7, the head of the family provided all income received during the year; in Family 6, the head of the household was a minor contributor to the family resources. In almost all families, however, women and children contribute something, however small, to the support of the family group.

Although the nuclear family is the basic economic group, more distant relatives often help each other with loans or gifts of money or goods when times are hard. "I don't know how we'd get by," Luisa said, "if it wasn't for my married daughter in Los Angeles. In the winter when my husband can't find work, she always sends a little money every time she gets a paycheck." Juana explained that her husband's brother had come to their assistance at a time when the family needed money badly: "Gilberto and I were having a pretty hard time then, so his brother said he would help us out —he didn't have any money to give, but he took the oldest boy to live with him for a while, bought all his food and some clothes for him for a few months."

Both relatives and nonrelatives assist each other through exchange of services. Paula "rented" one of her bedrooms to one of her friends, a widow, who helps Paula with her housework and laundry in exchange for the room. Ismael and his wife supplied board and room for several months to an elderly man, a pensioner, in exchange for gardening, yard work, and various "odd jobs" around the house. Alfonso and Rosa provided a home for Doña Clara, an elderly widow with no family of her own. "She lives here and helps Rosa with the housework," Alfonso said, "and we give her room and meals, buy her clothes, and take her with us wherever we go, like to the movies. It's good for us because Rosa needs someone to help with the housework, and I can take her off my income tax as another dependent. It's a good deal for everybody."

When other sources of income are inadequate for the provision of necessities, families attempt to borrow money from credit organizations or purchase goods on account. When the extension of credit fails, families seek public assistance from government agencies. The critical role played by credit in family economy is described in following pages.

EXPENDITURES

Long-range financial planning is not a customary procedure in Sal si Puedes. Budgeting is casual; during months when work is available and income is high, expenditures rise. In the winter season families seldom have money for more than the bare necessities of life. During the summer when wages are high there is a temptation to spend freely in order to acquire household goods and luxury items.

During the spring and summer of 1955, Ismael worked long hours and earned good wages, out of which he was able to save several hundred dollars—enough for a down payment on a new car. "If I don't buy the car now, something will happen to the money, and in the winter I couldn't afford to buy it," he said. Ismael bought the car in September, but when the first payment was due in October, Ismael's wife, Paula, complained: "I wasn't sure we should get a car this year, but Ismael wanted it so bad that I finally broke down and said okay. Now he's got the car, but I have to worry about the car payments—seventy-two dollars a month. We still have to pay the mortgage on the house, too. Now, with winter and bad weather coming, Ismael won't get to work every day, and when he doesn't work he doesn't get paid. It's going to be pretty hard now to make it through the winter without going more in debt."

Families who have higher incomes spend more money; the correlation of earning and spending is presented in table 7, showing estimates of annual expenditure of representative families in three income groups.

Generally, both the families of agricultural laborers and families of steadily employed workers live within their incomes. Industrial workers with seasonal employment, on the other hand, frequently spend more than they earn. A San Jose tax accountant, a Mexican-American himself, who helps a number of Mayfair families prepare their tax returns, reported: "Farm families like to pay their bills as they go along; they'd rather go without things they need than to go in debt too far. And people with year-round jobs are the same way. But the ones that get in the hole are the people that make high wages for part of the year and then get laid off in the winter—they get used to having money in their pockets and think they're rich. They go out and buy a lot of stuff on credit, and then when they get laid off, they can't meet the payments. They like to live a little better than the fruit pickers, and when their debts pile up, an appliance, a car, or a piece of furniture will have to be sold or repossessed to make up the difference." Of course, not all those who are steadily employed or who do farm work stay out of debt and not all seasonal industrial workers live beyond their means, but the tendency noted by the tax accountant was observed in the barrio.

TABLE 7

ANNUAL EXPENDITURES OF THREE SAL SI PUEDES FAMILIES

Expenditures	Seasonal farm worker's family	Seasonal nonfarm worker's family	Steadily employed worker's family
Housing: rent or payments, and repair	$ 600	$ 660	$ 900
Utilities	180	180	180
Food	900	1,200	1,500
Clothing	400	600	700
Time payments, except car	120	360	360
Transportation, car payments	420	420	840
Medical care, drugs, dentist	60	120	180
Contributions (church, relatives)	20	30	110
Insurance	—	—	120
Entertainment	200	300	360
Union Dues	—	40	50
Savings	—	—	80
Total expenditures	$2,900	$3,860	$4,500
Total income	2,900	3,600	4,500
Annual deficit	—	260	—

Families with either a little surplus capital or retail credit opportunities often purchase certain items which, according to some of their English-speaking neighbors, they "can't afford." One Anglo merchant commented on the number of television sets in Sal si Puedes: "Almost every house, even the poorest shack, has a television antenna." This statement is a slight exaggeration, but most families do own television sets, many of them rather elaborate console models. Consuela's house has limited sleeping facilities which require the children to sleep three to a bed, yet her kitchen boasts a magnificent new stove with two ovens, automatic timing devices, and a shining chromium top. Gilberto, whose two younger children had no shoes, bought a hundred dollars' worth of movie-camera equipment.

"The people here in east San Jose," commented a Spanish-speaking community worker, "enjoy buying certain 'luxury items' even if the expense means less money for groceries." Some of the things that people like to buy, he reported, are electric appliances, huge photographic portraits of family members, sets of encyclopedias, weather stripping or "insulation" for their homes, any sort of goods sold door to door, and insurance policies. "The weather stripping is usually wasted—it seals the windows, but cracks in the walls still let in the cold. They buy things that are sold door to door because they fall for high-pressure salesmanship and don't know how to say no. The insurance would be all right except that some people buy kinds they don't need,[4] sometimes get overlapping policies, and sometimes don't even collect the benefits because they don't understand the policies."

People spend a good deal of money on entertainment, sometimes as much as 10 or 15 per cent of their total income. Much of this money goes to purchase food and drink for the many parties and celebrations to which all relatives and friends are invited. Birthdays, bridal showers, wedding receptions, baby showers, "coming-out" parties for girls, and baptismal celebrations—all require the purchase of special foods to feed from twenty-five to two hundred guests. Some men in the neighborhood spend sizable sums of money on alcohol for themselves and for their friends.

The "uneconomical" purchasing patterns of many Sal si Puedes families leads people to believe in the popular theory that Mexican-Americans are financially irresponsible and improvident. Such a belief is not entirely justified, however. It seems unlikely that families of other ethnic backgrounds consistently resist the temptation to acquire coveted merchandise at the expense of other budgetary items. There are those who, regardless of cultural background, prefer to forego some of the more corporeal satisfactions in order to gain the spiritual rewards deriving from "luxuries" such as vacations

[4] Several Sal si Puedes families, for example, purchased "polio insurance" for their children. Of these families, some were eligible for hospital care at the county hospital and a few were already assured medical costs in the event of polio by general hospitalization coverage such as Blue Cross.

to Florida, new convertibles, or season tickets to the opera. The story of the stenographer who saved her lunch money to buy a new dress is not an unfamiliar one to most Anglos.

No doubt there are many reasons why barrio families purchase the things they do. A few of them are readily deduced: The values and demands of Mexican-American society, advertising and salesmanship, and the desire for social mobility are among the factors that influence buying patterns. Mexican-American culture places value on lavish entertainment of friends and relatives with food and drink; the emphasis on family life is reflected in the desire to have large portraits of family members. The desire to rise in the social class structure prompts people to acquire the commodities which advertising and salesmanship assure them are essential appurtenances of "the American way of life"—stoves, refrigerators, washing machines, insurance policies, weather stripping, and insulation. Doorto-door book salesmen find ready customers for sets of encyclopedias which parents proudly display as an indication that they value education for their children.

As Paula once said, "Nobody likes to be poor." In Sal si Puedes where so many people are struggling to escape poverty and want, a "luxury item" like a shiny new refrigerator may be the source of hope and encouragement—it may symbolize the first step toward the achievement of a better way of life.

CREDIT

Because so many of the people of Sal si Puedes have low incomes and are seasonally employed, the credit facilities open to them are somewhat limited.

One San Jose banker cautiously reported: "I can't say whether Mexicans as a group are good or bad risks—we deal with them on an individual basis." He added, however, "It's true that we might investigate Mexican loan prospects a little more thoroughly than someone else, but that's because so many are transients and others don't have steady jobs. If people don't provide ahead for slack work periods, they can't meet their payments."

Another banker, in discussing home-improvement loans, asserted that "some of the people live in slum areas, and home loans in those neighborhoods are considered special risks." Sal si Puedes, he said, is in one of those areas.

Although bank credit is available only to the few who have steady employment, retail stores are more liberal. There are several neighborhood grocery stores in Mayfair which extend credit to families during the winter months. Some seasonal workers may have grocery accounts of $200 to $400 at the end of the "slack season." During spring and summer, accounts are settled, and for a few months in late summer and fall, families can make cash purchases. But when the summer's savings are spent, seasonal workers are unemployed and must once more buy food on credit, and the cycle is repeated.

Groceries at neighborhood markets are slightly more expensive than at large supermarkets which operate on a cash basis. For this reason, those who can afford to pay cash for their supplies prefer to shop at supermarkets.

Families who have periods of unemployment worry about possible loss of credit. If a family loses the good will of the neighborhood storekeeper, there may be winter days when the children go to school with stomachs half-empty. A neighbor told of Inez's credit problems: "She made a mistake and told the man at the store that her husband got paid regularly. I guess she wanted to be sure he'd give them the credit. But then her husband got laid off, and when the bill got behind, the man cut off her credit. Now she is looking for credit at another store, and I guess they need it pretty bad right now because Inez is borrowing flour and beans from her comadre."

In 1954 a step was taken toward solving credit problems for the Spanish-speaking people of east San Jose by the formation of a credit union. It was organized at the suggestion of the priest of the Chapel of Our Lady of Guadalupe, but membership was nonsectarian. One of the members described the formation of the union: "At first there were just eleven members, and we had only five hundred dollars when we got our charter. At first it was slow getting started because the people didn't understand what a credit union was. Most of them thought it was a sort of church bank and that the priest was lending people money. Some people were afraid because they didn't trust the officers and thought they would lose their money. Finally, after the priest explained about it in church a few times, people began to join."

In a year's time the credit union had approximately a hundred members. By the end of 1955, a total of about seventy-five loans had been made, most of them to members who needed money for down payments on homes. Some loans were made for the purchase of automobiles or furniture and a few were personal loans. Maximum credit extended to a single member was $300. Of all loans made up until that time, only one had proved impossible to collect and necessitated court action. At the end of 1955, total deposits were approximately $4,000, and success of the project seemed assured.

ASSETS AND PROPERTY

A relatively large number, 62 per cent, of Sal si Puedes families own their homes. Houses are typically four- or five-room frame dwellings on lots measuring 40 by 100 feet. Most homes in 1955 had a retail market value of $4,000 to $5,000. County tax assessment evaluations were considerably lower, averaging between $1,000 and $2,000.

The people dislike paying rent and place considerable emphasis on the advantages of home ownership. Ramón, a former barrio resident, bought a new home in 1954. "I had a lot of trouble renting houses," he explained. "There were so many landlords that wouldn't rent to people with kids, and for fifty dollars a month you couldn't get more than a shack. For a decent house in a nice neighborhood I would have to pay seventy-five or eighty dollars a month—at those prices, you are just working for the landlord." Since the advent of the neighborhood credit union in 1954, there is opportunity for an increasing number of families to buy homes. This tendency may not be reflected in the proportion of home owners in the neighborhood, however, because some families move into new homes in other districts. Frequently, former residents of the barrio retain their holdings there as income property.

Movable assets of neighborhood families are mainly household furnishings, personal effects, and family cars. Three men own pickup trucks, and several families have house trailers.

Assets in the form of savings or investments are rare. About a dozen families own a few shares in the credit union, but individual holdings average less than $100. About a third of the families have insurance policies, most of which are burial insurance or low-premium life policies with little cash value. The factory workers usually have medical-insurance coverage through group hospitalization plans at their place of employment, but seasonal laborers, with rare exceptions, lack medical coverage.

The people of Sal si Puedes, living as they do so near the edge of poverty, "cannot afford" to be sick. For most of them a serious illness requiring prolonged hospitalization is a financial catastrophe. In spite of economic problems, however, barrio people look back on the deprivations of earlier years and take heart from the increased resources they now have. They make the best of things, remain cheerful, and hope for better times to come.

5

THE PATTERN OF RELIGIOUS LIFE

CUSTOM AND belief concerning man's relation to the supernatural affect phases of life, and are of particular significance to people in times of crisis, especially when some danger appears to threaten life or health. For this reason Mexican-American religious beliefs and practices are of more than academic interest to those who meet Spanish-speaking people in medical situations.

Religious belief and ceremony play an important part in the lives of Mayfair residents, but the role of religion in that community is not identical with its function in either Mexican societies or Anglo communities. Religious belief and church organizations are perhaps significantly more potent forces in Mayfair than in Anglo sections of San Jose. But the religious complex in Mexican-American life is not the all-pervading influence that it is said to be in the villages of Jalisco, Michoacán, and Guanajuato from which so many Mexican-Americans or their parents emigrated.[1]

The aspects of Mexican-American religious life which are of particular interest to public health workers are: (1) the role of religious groups in community solidarity or social differentiation; (2) the influence of the churches on the acceptance or rejection of Anglo cultural patterns by Spanish-speaking people; and (3) the functions of religion in community life and its effect on individual behavior.

RELIGIOUS SECTS

Religious affiliation of Spanish-speaking people in Mayfair community as a whole and in the barrio of Sal si Puedes were as follows in 1955: [2]

Religious preference	Mayfair community		Sal si Puedes	
	Number	Per cent	Number	Per cent
Catholic	2,247	70.6	370	87.6
Protestant	810	25.4	32	7.7
No preference	126	4.0	20	4.7
Total	3,183	100.0	422	100.0

Sal si Puedes obviously is overwhelmingly Catholic. Mayfair is strongly Catholic, but the Protestants (as pointed out in chapter 2) constitute about one-fourth of the total population. Most Protestants are members of Pentecostal sects, two of which have churches in Mayfair. A few families are Baptists and a slightly larger number are Seventh-Day Adventists. There was a Baptist church in Sal si Puedes until 1954, but since that time the church building has been vacant, the congregation occupying another building in San Jose proper. There is a Seventh-Day Adventist church in Los Calles barrio, and several of its congregation live in that neighborhood. The Methodists have a small mission for Spanish-speaking people in

[1] Religious beliefs and practices of Mexican villagers have been recorded by a number of writers. Some of them are: Parsons, [34], pp. 183–315; Beals [3], 116–163; Foster, [16], pp. 188–224; and Toor, [47].

[2] The data in the table are from two sources. Those for Mayfair are based on a 20 per cent sample of Mexican-Americans registered in a community health survey in November, 1955; those for Sal si Puedes were derived from a two-thirds sample of all families of the barrio surveyed in an ethnographic census taken in April, 1955. The figures agree closely with information supplied by Mayfair Elementary School authorities, who report approximately the same Catholic-Protestant ratio among their school population.

San Jose, but its membership is drawn principally from areas out-side the Mayfair District.

Since most Mayfair families are Catholic, the following discussion of religious life is weighted in favor of descriptions of Catholic ceremony and belief.

Sharp social divisions along sectarian lines separate the people of Mayfair community into religious factions. "There are too many religions here," Ramón commented. "I think the people would be better organized if there was only one church; and people don't like a person who belongs to another church—they gossip and talk about each other and pretty soon there's a lot of trouble."

Catholic clergymen and Protestant ministers of Mexican-American churches in the area are all willing to support community projects which they regard as generally beneficial. However, attempts to arrange meetings of Catholic and Protestant clergymen for co-operative planning have not always been successful.[3]

Relations between Catholics and Protestants in Mayfair are less cordial than those between members of a single religious group. Ismael, who is active in the Catholic church, reported, "My wife and I used to have some very good friends that we had known for years. We used to visit with them a lot and have good times together. Then a couple of years ago these friends joined a Pen-tecostal church, and right after that they stopped coming to see us. I guess it was because we smoke and drink a little beer and go to parties. Their church teaches that having fun is a sin, and I guess they thought it was wrong to be friends with us any more."

A Protestant resident of McCreery barrio commented: "We've tried to be friendly with our next-door neighbors, the Padilla family, but Mrs. Padilla is such a strong Catholic that she makes us feel uncomfortable—she keeps shaking her head and telling us that our parents would be ashamed of us for turning our backs on our religion. I try to tell her that my family has been Protestant for three generations, but she doesn't believe me."

In spite of the social division along sectarian lines, individuals of

[3] For example, members of the county public health department reported that efforts to arrange a meeting of Catholic and Protestant clergymen to plan a pub-licity campaign for a community X-ray survey were unsuccessful, although all the ministers approached were willing to coöperate directly with representatives of the health department. Three of the Protestant ministers, however, did attend a joint planning session.

different religious beliefs may be close friends. Manuela, a Catholic, described how she and her family spent Thanksgiving Day: "We had dinner with some of our friends in town who used to live in our barrio. They are Baptists, but they are good friends and we had a nice day."

Consuela said of a Protestant neighbor, "I don't know her very well because she's a holiness church woman—but she seems like a very nice lady, anyway."

CATHOLICISM

Mayfair's Catholic church, the Chapel of Our Lady of Guadalupe, was built in 1952. Grounds and building materials were purchased by the bishop of San Francisco, but much of the labor of constructing the building was done by members of the local community.

Before 1948 there were no Catholic services held in Mayfair, and Mexican-American Catholics in the community either attended other churches in San Jose or, more commonly, did not attend mass at all except perhaps on special occasions. Paula, commenting on the Mayfair Catholic community before 1948, said, "Some of our people didn't feel comfortable in those American churches—they didn't feel like they were very welcome there, so lots of times they just didn't go to church. Then the Protestants started coming around and inviting the people to go to their churches. Plenty of times they tried to get me to go, and if the fathers hadn't come about that time, we would all be *Protestantes* now!"

In 1948 the Catholics acquired a building in Sal si Puedes, a small public hall formerly owned by a Mexican-American burial society. There, from 1948 to 1952, Catholic services were held once a month by an Anglo priest. In 1952 the Mayfair District was classified by the Catholic diocese as a mission area, and a Spanish-speaking Anglo missionary priest was assigned to work full time in the community. The new priest was instrumental in obtaining funds for a new church building. When the new building, the Chapel of Our Lady of Guadalupe, was completed in December, 1952, the small hall was converted into a youth center.

The Chapel is a stucco structure, topped by a squat belfry; the floor plan is cruciform, and seating for about 250 people is provided. Anterooms include a baptistry and a sacristy which also serves as the church office. Behind the altar hangs a large image of Christ on the Cross, and on either side stand figures of *santos*. A large picture of the Virgin of Guadalupe, the patroness of Mexico, occupies a prominent place above the altar. A small image of *El Santo Niño de Atocha* (the Holy Child of Atocha), a Spanish saint who is regarded with particular reverence by Guadalupe parishioners, stands near the right transept.

In 1955 four masses, each with an average attendance of about 175, were held each Sunday at the Chapel. As many as 1,200 people, many of them from other parts of the colony, sometimes came to mass on special days. The Anglo priest celebrates most masses, usually conducting the non-Latin parts of the service in Spanish. The people of the parish often comment on their good fortune in having a padre who, although non-Mexican, speaks Spanish so well. Aside from the fact that sermons are in Spanish, services differ from the usual Anglo ritual in that a lay reader stands to one side of the altar and translates each Latin passage into Spanish.

CHURCH ORGANIZATION

Since the Chapel was erected, four auxiliary societies have been organized by parishioners: a girls' catechism class, an altar boys' society, an older girls' choir, and a women's altar society. Of these, the largest and most active is the Altar Society, the Sociedad Guadalupana; its members clean the church building, maintain altar accessories and vestments, and raise money for church improvements. To one side of the Chapel a small frame hut was built by the Sociedad Guadalupana; it is used as a kitchen and food stand by the women of the group who raise money by selling and serving Mexican foods there after mass each Sunday. The Sociedad is particularly concerned with the celebration of the Fiesta of the Virgin of Guadalupe on December 12.

The men of the Catholic congregation have no formal organization. A group of ten or twelve men of the community, however, keep all-night vigils at the Chapel on the first Friday of each month, rotating in groups of two or three.

About eighteen months before this study began, a Catholic youth center was organized. The small hall in Sal si Puedes was provided with athletic and recreational equipment, and a young man of another parish was selected to sponsor the group. Within a year, however, interest in the youth program began to lag, and the only remnant of the program remaining was an occasional evening of amateur boxing. A few months later the entire recreation program was abandoned, and the hall was no longer used.

Catholic people in the community had various explanations for the failure of the program. One explanation was that there was an initial surge of interest on the part of boys in the community, but then some who had been interested only in the novelty began to stop coming. The sponsor tried to rekindle flagging local interest by bringing in outsiders—boys from other parishes were invited to participate in boxing matches and other athletic events. "There got to be so many outsiders," one parishioner remarked, "that the people here felt like the youth center didn't belong to them anymore." Other observers believed that the boys of the community were interested in the center until the sponsor accepted a job as a juvenile probation officer. "People say that when he took that police job the neighborhood boys didn't trust him anymore—they thought he was just another cop and was only working at the center to keep them in line."

In February, 1955, an attempt was made by local Catholic leaders to reorganize the youth group. This attempt got no further than preliminary discussion, however. A controversy arose between members of the planning committee over whether or not the center should be open to non-Catholics. Ten months later, when the research for this book was completed, no decision had been reached, and the youth center was apparently defunct. The case of the youth center illustrates some of the problems of leadership and factionalism which defeat attempts to initiate community programs. Health programs are not immune to difficulties of this kind.

Church organization at the Chapel is essentially Anglo-American in form. Many features of Mexican Catholic organization are absent; for example, a women's altar society takes over duties ordinarily performed in Mexican village churches by *cargueros*, men responsible for the care of images of the saints. There are clubs and a credit union for Mayfair Catholics, but no formally organized group of parishioners in charge of religious celebrations. In the details of ceremonial practice, however, Mexican patterns are much in evidence.

CEREMONIAL CALENDAR

Religious practice among Mayfair Catholics actually consists of three separate ceremonial systems rather than a single integrated form.

The core of religious life is formed by the traditional rituals of the Church of Rome which are the responsibility of the priest and his assistants. In this category are the rosary and the various sacraments (mass, baptism, communion, confirmation, confession). A second aspect of religious practice is a group of ceremonials based on Catholicism but conducted primarily by lay members of the community. The priest may be called upon to play a part in some of these rituals, but others are performed entirely by laymen. These ceremonies are discussed in the following pages. Miscellaneous religious beliefs and customs which are individual, rather than group, activities constitute a third aspect of religious behavior. It is in the two latter aspects of religion that Mexican patterns are most apparent.

For Mexican-American Catholics in Mayfair, the ceremonial year revolves around the Christmas season, the Easter season, and the Fiesta of the Virgin of Guadalupe, patroness of the local church. Highlights of this annual cycle follow.

Día de los Santos Reyes, January 6 (Epiphany): The Day of the Holy Kings commemorates the visit of the Magi to the Christ Child. In many parts of Mexico it is an occasion for special festivities [40]. In San Jose in 1955, the day was a purely secular one, with a benefit dance at a public ballroom in downtown San Jose. The benefit was sponsored by two Mexican-American civic groups (welfare committee of the *Commisión Honorífica Mexicana* and the San Jose Mexican Chamber of Commerce), and proceeds from the dance were used to buy food and clothing for distribution to needy families of the San Jose Spanish-speaking colony.

Day of San Antonio, January 17: The blessing of domestic animals on the feast of San Antonio, a Catholic tradition in Mexico, was first inaugurated by the priest of the Chapel in 1955 at the request of a group of parishioners. People of the community brought chickens, dogs, cats, and rabbits to the churchyard to be blessed by the priest.

La Candelaria, February 2 (Candlemas): Candlemas was observed with a mass, followed by the blessing of candles to be used during the year when a religious observance was held in the home or to be burned during the last rites administered to a dying person.

Day of San Blas, February 3: Following mass at the Chapel there was a blessing of throats by the priest. (San Blas is the patron of throat ailments.) The priest crossed two long candles which he held in his hands and surrounded each parishioner's throat with one of the angles formed by the cross.

Lent: Although in 1954 a number of Mexican Lenten ceremonials were introduced at the Chapel, Mayfair Catholics generally felt that the season was insufficiently celebrated in San Jose. Tomasa commented, "It's a pity that the Mexican people here have lost most of their religious customs, especially the ones for *La Cuaresma* (Lent). All of us who are from Mexico remember the carnivals in our villages." Carnival is not observed in Mayfair although some families have private parties in their homes just before Lent.

Ash Wednesday: On the first day of Lent the people came for confession and to have their foreheads marked with a cross of ashes by the priest. The ashes were obtained from burned palm fronds which had been saved from the previous year's Palm Sunday procession.

Six Fridays of Lent: On each of the Friday evenings of Lent, the people came to the Chapel to say a rosary and visit each of the pictures representing the Fourteen Stations of the Cross. There was no other ceremony.

Palm Sunday: On Saturday before Palm Sunday, palm branches were collected and taken to the Chapel to be used to decorate the interior for mass on the following day. After mass the priest blessed the palms by sprinkling them with holy water, and they were then distributed to members of the congregation. Some used strips of palm leaf to form small crosses which were tacked over doorways of homes to protect family members from illness or other harm. Occasionally pieces of the blessed palm were used in curing rites (see chapter 7).

Good Friday: Mass was scheduled at twelve noon. All the images and holy pictures in the church except those representing the Stations of the Cross were draped with purple cloth. The priest, assisted by two novices, said mass. At intervals he stopped while a lay reader repeated through a public address system a brief Spanish translation of the Latin ritual which had just preceded.

During mass the large image of Christ on the Cross was divested of its purple draperies. A little later a smaller crucifix which had stood on the main altar was taken down by one of the novices and laid on a purple satin cushion on the floor in front of the altar, a procedure symbolizing the descent from the Cross.

Following mass the priest preached a short sermon in Spanish dealing with the doctrine of atonement. Following that he delivered the traditional "Sermon of the Seven Words." The service concluded at three o'clock.

On the evening of Good Friday the people once more gathered at the Chapel for the *Vía Crucis* ("Way of the Cross"), a traditional Mexican observance held in San Jose for the first time in 1954. Several members of the Sociedad Guadalupana (Altar Society) passed through the congregation distributing candles for the procession. In front of the church the people formed a procession, led by two torchbearers. The priest followed, walking just ahead of a large wooden cross carried by about twenty men. The cross, made out of a telephone pole, was about twenty-five feet long and about eight feet across—evidently a tremendous weight because the bearers staggered under the load. Additional torchbearers and the ladies of the Sociedad Guadalupana with tricolored sashes over their shoulders followed the cross. The rest of the congregation followed carrying lighted candles which they cupped in their hands to shield the guttering flames from the night wind. The procession moved down the dark street to a vacant field nearby. There was no music and no singing, but some of the people murmured prayers as they walked along. In the field thirteen small white wooden crosses about four feet high were set up at about thirty foot intervals around three sides of the area. At the fourth side a large mound of dirt about eight feet in height had been piled up to represent *Calvario,* or Calvary, which was the last or fourteenth Station of the Cross. The procession moved from one cross to the next and finally the large cross was set in a deep hole on top of the Calvario, where it was left until the next day.

The procession was a curious amalgamation of Mexican and American elements: women with silk scarves or shawls over their heads and men in their Sunday suits moved in silent procession, their lips reciting prayers in Spanish, their faces glowing in the light of the candles they held, following the dark torch-lit bulk of the massive cross. But strangely mixed with these elements there were the glare of flashbulbs, the voice of the padre blaring out of a loudspeaker, and, a few blocks away, the flashing neon of supermarkets and the roar of heavy diesel trucks hauling valley produce toward San Francisco.

Sábado de Gloria (Easter Saturday): At the Chapel in 1955, the

Misa de Gloria (Easter Mass) was scheduled to begin about ten thirty Saturday night. In the United States this is the approximate time regularly set aside. In Mexico, however, the mass celebrating the end of Lent is usually said Saturday morning. In 1955, when it was announced that Easter would be celebrated at the Chapel with a midnight mass, many of the parishioners felt that they had been cheated out of a day's celebration by the prolonging of the Lenten season for an extra day. "Some of us went to talk to Father about that," Marta said, "but he still wouldn't change the time. Of course Father is better than he used to be about our traditions. The people have talked to him a lot about Mexican ways; he has helped us bring back some of our customs, but there are still a lot of things that the people would like that he doesn't approve of."

The Easter service began about eleven o'clock Saturday night with the blessing of holy water to be used for various purposes during the following year. The ritual was performed by a visiting Anglo priest (not the regular padre) and two assistants. After the water was blessed the priest had all the candles in the church extinguished, made new fire (lit a special paschal or Easter candle with a match), blessed the fire, and had all other candles lit from it.

A high mass followed these ceremonies. At the close of the Misa de Gloria, the priest spoke briefly in Spanish, announcing that Judas would be burned in the churchyard after the service.

The "burning of Judas," a widespread Mexican Easter custom, was revived at the Chapel in 1954 at the request of some of the parishioners. Consuela, a well-known seamstress, had made a life size *mono*, a dummy representing Judas, which she dressed in American street clothing—gray suit, socks, shoes, and felt hat. The hands were formed by cotton gloves, and the head was of cloth painted with a face, the most striking feature of which was a huge black handle-bar mustache. The over-all effect was that of a caricature of the villain in a "Gay Nineties" melodrama.

This effigy was suspended in the churchyard. Following mass, the priest set fire to it, igniting the firecrackers and sparklers with which it was stuffed and adorned. The pyrotechnic display, although less elaborate than those of Mexico, was felt to be highly gratifying to all participants. As in Mexico, Easter Sunday had no special ritual other than the usual mass.

Anniversary of the founding of the Chapel of Our Lady of Guada-

lupe, October 9: In 1955 the members of the Chapel celebrated the third anniversary of its founding with a procession and a jamaica (church bazaar and carnival, similar to that described below in connection with the Fiesta of the Virgin of Guadalupe). The principal function of the fiesta seemed to be to raise money for the church.

Fiesta of the Virgin of Guadalupe, December 12: The Virgin of Guadalupe is the patroness of the Indians of Mexico and also of the Chapel in Mayfair. The annual festival held in her honor is the most elaborate Catholic fiesta held at the Chapel during the year.

The ceremonies and festivities of the day are the special province of the women of the Sociedad Guadalupana, whose members are particularly devoted to the Virgin of Guadalupe. They make most of the plans and preparations for the fiesta, and press their husbands and other men of the church into helping them with the heavy work. Two or three weeks before time for the fiesta, members of the Sociedad were busy soliciting donations or making objects (embroidery, crocheted doilies) to be sold or given as prizes during the jamaica which was to be a part of the celebration. The day before the fiesta, several men of the parish erected in the churchyard a series of wooden booths to be used as food stands or game concessions. Other members of the Sociedad and their husbands were inside the church making last-minute preparations. The large image of Christ on the Cross which ordinarily hung directly behind the main altar had been removed, and the painting of the Virgin of Guadalupe placed there instead.

Early on the morning of December 12 (which in 1954 fell on a Sunday), the fiesta began with *las mañanitas,* a special mass in honor of the Virgin. During the morning, one of the food stands was open and a number of people gathered to eat menudo (Mexican tripe) and drink coffee. The procession began at noon about two blocks from the church. The group was led by two young girls in *China Poblana* costumes carrying a small banner depicting the Virgin. About eight Mexican-American men in American Legion uniforms followed carrying the American and Mexican flags. Then came about a dozen young girls in white dresses with crepe-paper wings; they were led by a "queen," a little girl about six years old who rode in a small cart pulled by two men. The child was dressed to represent the Virgin of Guadalupe. Following the "angels" in the procession were two men bearing the main banner with the picture of the Virgin. Behind the banner marched a group of children, some small girls in white confirmation dresses carrying arches decorated with green paper and yellow roses, others dressed as *charros* and "Spanish ladies," some older girls in China Problana costume, and several boys in Indian costumes. Some of these represented Juan Diego, the Mexican Indian to whom the Virgin appeared miraculously, and others were dressed as "Apaches," or wild Indians, with feather headdresses, breechcloths, and bare bellies and legs. A group of men and women parishioners ended the procession. When the procession reached the church, the people entered and another mass was said.

Meanwhile, outside in the churchyard, jazz records were played over a loudspeaker, families bought Mexican food at the booths (tamales, tacos, menudo, Spanish rice, enchiladas, coffee, and soft drinks), and play started at the various "game booths," including a bingo game and a *ruleta,* or "wheel of fortune," which gave pigeons and roosters as prizes. Other funds were raised by means of "deputy sheriffs" with silver stars, who "arrested" people on flimsy charges such as putting their hands in their pockets. Those who were "arrested" paid small "fines." Business was quite brisk for a while.

There was some dancing to phonograph records (in 1955 a more elaborate musical program was supplied by two groups of Mexican-American musicians hired for the jamaica), and a program of music, folk dancing, and recitations. The fiesta ended with a rosary at 7:00 P.M.

Las Posadas (The Lodgings), December 16–24: The *Posadas* depict the journey of Mary and Joseph to Bethlehem and their search for lodgings. For nine nights before Christmas these little ceremonies take place. In Mexico they are generally affairs in which relatives and friends cooperate and in which both adults and children participate. Mexican posadas are generally given at a different house every night, and always terminate with the breaking of a *piñata,* a clay jar filled with candy and toys.

In Mayfair the posadas are attended almost exclusively by women and children. The ceremony consisted of a rosary at one house, followed by a procession to another home of the community. The procession was led by two children carrying a small litter which held two figurines representing Mary and Joseph. About twenty women and children followed the litter, carrying lighted candles and singing. When they arrived at the house that was their destination, one of the "pilgrims" in the procession knocked at the door, to be told (in the form of a song) by those inside the house that there was "no room at the inn." After more singing, the door was opened, and the marchers went inside, deposited the litter with the saints near the family altar, said some prayers, and had refreshments. The children were given candy and nuts, sometimes chocolate and fruit, and the women sipped cups of Mexican chocolate and chatted with their friends. There was no piñata, however. This ceremony was repeated each evening until Christmas Eve.

Los Pastores (The Shepherds): A *pastorela*, or Christmas pageant, was given in Mayfair in 1954, the first time such a presentation had been given in the community. The particular version of *Los Pastores* used was brought from a village in Sonora, Mexico, by a San Jose woman who had been born and reared there. She had made a *manda*, or promise, to the Virgin of Guadalupe to sponsor a production of the pageant just as it was given in her home village in Mexico. When it came time to fulfill the vow, she had trouble because there was no written copy of it in existence that she could find. She wrote to her village and arranged for the local school-teacher there to take down the words in dictation from some of the villagers. In this way, an oral tradition of a small Mexican village was transported to a suburban community of northern California.

The pageant was much like traditional Mexican pastorelas, with shepherds, angels, an old hermit, a devil, and, for a comic touch, an Indian who insisted on going to Bethlehem to offer the Christ Child a plate of enchiladas. The play was followed by mass and communion at midnight on Christmas Eve, and was the last ritual event of the Catholic ceremonial year in Mayfair.

INDIVIDUAL RELIGIOUS ACTIVITIES

Most Mexican-American Catholics in Mayfair observe the principal sacraments of the church: they are baptized, confirmed, married, and buried with Catholic rites. At each of these ceremonial events, except burial, the person is sponsored by godparents, or *padrinos*, who thus become coparents, or compadres, of his own mother and father. (The system of formalized social relationships between compadres is discussed in chapter 6.)

About half of the Catholic homes visited in Mayfair had a small shrine or altar in some corner of the house. A fairly representative one, in Carmen's living room, was simply a small shelf (of the type sometimes sold in American variety stores for bric-a-brac), above which was a picture of the Virgin of Guadalupe bordered with artificial flowers. On the shelf were a small statue of El Santo Niño de Atocha, a crucifix, and two votive lights. Tacked to the wall on either side of the shelf were miniature American and Mexican flags and various religious cards and medals.

A number of Catholics in Mayfair from time to time make mandas, or vows, to a particular saint or Virgin which they promise to keep in exchange for a favor. For example, when Amelia's oldest daughter was hospitalized for tuberculosis, Amelia made a promise to the Virgin of San Juan de los Lagos that if her daughter recovered she would visit the town of San Juan de los Lagos in Mexico and make an offering at the shrine there. When her daughter was discharged from the sanatorium, Amelia saved money for three years and finally acquired enough capital to fulfill the vow. Another Guadalupe parishioner, Antonio, made a manda to the Virgin of Guadalupe when he was in the U. S. Army during World War II. For several years he was unable to fulfill the vow, but finally in 1952 he and his wife made a trip to the shrine of the Virgin at La Villa de Guadalupe near Mexico City, where Antonio lit a candle to the Virgin and bought and hung votive offerings (silver arms, legs, and other parts of the body) in the appropriate places in the church there. "In war time," Antonio remarked, "when you were afraid, you thought of trying anything, and making a manda seemed like a good idea. A lot of Mexican boys made that promise, but most of them forgot about it when they got home safe and very few ever went to Mexico."

In the making of vows and offerings, barrio people usually give preference to Virgins and saints who have Spanish or Mexican connections. Thus travelers or truck drivers usually pray to El Santo Niño de Atocha for safe journeys rather than to St. Christopher, usually thought of by Catholics as the patron of travelers. Local priests sometimes try to encourage a shift of emphasis from purely Mexican religious figures, but they have little success.

In this and in some other respects Mexican-American Catholics find that their religious beliefs and practices do not coincide with the emphases of the Catholic Church in the United States. For example, the priest at the Chapel objected to the presentation of the Christmas pastorela because, he said, "In the parts of Mexico where these plays were given there are very few priests, and the village usually has no Christmas Mass or communion. In those villages the people have developed certain rituals like the pastorela to take the place of mass. But here in the United States, where we have all the rituals of the church, it's ridiculous to have a ceremony which was designed to replace the mass." In spite of the absence of official sanction for certain of these individual religious observances of Mexican origin, there is still considerable emphasis placed on them by many Chapel parishioners.

A large body of magical belief and practice of Catholic derivation forms a part of diagnosis and home treatment of disease in Mayfair. The use of fragments of holy palm taken from the church on Palm Sunday has been mentioned above. There is wide incorporation of prayers and religious invocations in spells designed to cure a variety of disorders, particularly those thought to be magical in origin. Religious mementos and ceremonial objects are also used in ways which will be more fully described in chapter 7.

RELIGIOUS ATTITUDES

The priest of the Chapel and his assistants have made a concerted effort to establish a full Catholic ritual in Mayfair. This effort began in 1952 with the founding of the Chapel, and from that time to the present a number of inactive Catholic families have been encouraged to participate in church activities. Before the Catholic Church began its mission program in Mayfair, there were few families who took part in religious activities other than attending mass infrequently and having their babies baptized.

In 1955 about 35 to 40 per cent of Mayfair Catholics attended church fairly regularly, and about 20 to 25 per cent were active in church affairs.[4] Although most of them are only nominal Catholics, they preserve the rudiments of their faith, in having their children baptized in the church, keeping an image of the Virgin of Guadalupe somewhere in the house, and making certain that a dying person receives the last rites from a priest.

Those who attend church regularly are a small percentage of the

[4] These estimates are based on reports from Catholic leaders in the community and confirmed by my own observations.

total Catholic group, mainly women, older men, and young children. Only a handful of men attend the Chapel regularly, and adolescents and young adults generally are not very interested in religious activities. Young Catholic parents, however, do send their children to catechism classes and encourage them to receive religious instruction and be confirmed. Not all Catholic parents insist on this, however; one mother remarked: "My oldest son is sixteen now but he's never been confirmed. I had him baptized, but when he got a little older he said he didn't care about all that church business, so I didn't make him go. I figure it's up to him now to make up his own mind if he wants to go to church." A man in the community who has a teen-age son was discussing the problems of Mexican-American boys in San Jose. He said, "I get so tired of everybody who tries to work with these kids harping on the church all the time; the problem will never be solved that way. You can't appeal to the younger generation through religion any more; they just aren't interested in it—they are looking for something practical."

Mayfair Catholic children attend services, but adults of the parish complain that the children do not "take the Church seriously" and are undisciplined at religious gatherings. The general lack of pious behavior of which adults complain was evident during the Via Crucis procession on Good Friday. A group of boys about eight to twelve years old ran around through the gathered people, shouting, laughing, and playing with burning sticks. They took turns sliding down the side of the "Calvary" on the seats of their trousers, and in general seemed to have a wonderful time.

For those who are casual in their Catholic beliefs, religion is not a very significant force, but although they have little interest in religious activities they retain a nominal connection with the church and attend mass occasionally. The other 35 to 40 per cent of Mayfair Catholics are fervent in their beliefs; for them religion is a part of everyday life, a vital force which influences much of their behavior. They find in the church a source of spiritual guidance, a place of recreation, and a means of establishing friendly social relationships with other Catholic families of similar inclination.

PROTESTANTISM

Mexican-American Protestant churches in the San Jose area are generally of two types: possessional (of the "spirit") and nonpossessional sects. Nonpossessional Protestants are affiliated with four churches of three denominations in San Jose: one Methodist, one Seventh-Day Adventist, and two Baptist churches. All have Mexican-American ministers and have services conducted in Spanish. These churches are patterned closely after their Anglo counterparts in organization, doctrine, and ritual.

Spanish-speaking Methodists and Baptists in Mayfair are generally from Texas or New Mexico, where active mission programs were established among Spanish-speaking people during the years of heavy Mexican immigration following the Mexican Revolution of 1910. Few of these Protestants are direct converts from Catholicism, but are children of parents who became Protestants during their early years in the United States. The Seventh-Day Adventists in Mayfair, however, are an actively proselyting group. They acquired most of their membership in the early 1950's during an intensive canvassing and visiting campaign in Mayfair.

A second and much larger group of Protestants is affiliated with eight Mexican-American churches of Pentecostal, or "Holiness," type. These are actively proselyting sects characterized by some form of spirit possession. There are two Pentecostal churches in Mayfair.

One of these, the Latin-American Assembly of God church is an adobe-brick building constructed in 1954 about one block from the Chapel of Our Lady of Guadalupe. The auditorium is undecorated except for four large Gothic arches between which are set high windows of amber translucent glass. The platform is bordered by a kneeling board running the full length of the chancel, and holds a pulpit, three high-backed chairs, banners of two church auxiliaries, and an American flag. Anterooms are a vestibule and four Sunday school classrooms. The building of the Apostolic Church of Faith in Jesus Christ is somewhat older than the Assembly of God structure, but is of the same general pattern.

The two Pentecostal congregations are about equal in membership, each having a weekly attendance of seventy-five to one hundred persons usually and about two hundred on special occasions such as Easter and Christmas. Both hold morning and evening church services and prayer meetings one or two evenings during the week.

San Jose observers have several theories to explain the relatively large numbers of Spanish-speaking families in east San Jose who have been converted to Protestantism. A Catholic priest in the area said, "Protestant churches were successful largely because there was no active Catholic program for the Spanish-speaking people. Religion for the people there had never been a very personal experience, and the intense emotionalism of the more fervent groups, such as the Pentecostal sects, had great appeal for them. Also, the Protestants began active mission programs in Mayfair in the 1930's and 1940's." The Mexican-American Methodist minister in San Jose had much the same explanation for the change in religious allegiance of many Mayfair people, but added another comment: "Another factor in the Protestant trend may be that the Mexican people find themselves surrounded by Protestant Americans. I think that becoming Protestant represented to many Mexican-Americans a way of becoming better assimilated into Anglo life, and not being 'foreign' any more."

The Pentecostal sects of Mayfair are strict in their definitions of morality. Indulgence in tobacco, alcohol, dancing, and card playing are considered sinful. The pastor of one church also preaches that women should never cut their hair. Dora, a member of that congregation, commented, "Our church is pretty strict and not many people are willing to pay the price of following such a strict religion, but we believe that it's the right way and we know that it has its rewards."

CHURCH ORGANIZATION

The three Protestant denominations of Mayfair community are similar in organization; therefore only one, the Latin-American Assembly of God, will be described in detail.

The minister of the church is a second-generation Mexican-American who conducts services in Spanish. Because church congregations have a large proportion of older members who speak only Spanish, there is little chance of Mayfair people taking an active interest in a church in which services are conducted in English. Language is too great a barrier for most Mexican-American churchgoers. The success of Protestant church programs (and perhaps Catholic ones, too) depends on the availability of Spanish-speaking ministers. (This fact indicates the importance of language in community programs.)

Responsibility for the operation of the church rests with a board of deacons which meets from time to time with the minister. Other church organizations at the Assembly of God are a women's auxiliary whose duty is the maintenance of the church building and yard, a number of Sunday school classes, a youth group, and a choir of older girls.

The Baptist church which moved from Mayfair to downtown San Jose in 1954 once sponsored a boy scout troop, but the organization was not successful. One member of that congregation attributed the failure of the scout troop to poor leadership: "Nobody would stick with the boys for very long at a time. At first a scoutmaster would get all steamed up, but then he'd get tired of the job and quit. Sometimes I think you can't depend on Mexican leaders to take charge of Mexican groups—they lose their enthusiasm too fast."

One of the Mayfair Pentecostal churches has a group known as *Los de Don* (Those with the Gift). It was described as "a special group of people who have meetings every Saturday night to pray for people who are sick. Sometimes they will go to the homes of sick people and pray at their bedsides. Their job is mainly to cure people by faith." Mary, another member of the congregation, related what happened when she discovered she had tuberculosis: "Right away the people at our church began to have prayer meetings for me; they were held by a special group of people whose job is to pray for the sick to be healed. Of course, I know that those people didn't heal me because you can be cured only by faith. But they did pray for me to have more faith so I would be healed. I guess it worked because I'm getting well, and nobody here at the hospital is doing anything for me."

CHURCH ACTIVITIES

Pentecostal church groups have many activities for their parishioners: there are Sunday school classes, a summer Bible school for children, weekly youth meetings, two church services every Sunday, one or two prayer meetings a week, rallies, choir rehearsals, church picnics and dinners, and meetings of various church auxiliaries. Pentecostal groups have as one of their principal characteristics the phenomenon of "possession by the Holy Spirit," which distinguishes them from other Christian sects, both Catholic and Protestant. The experience of "possession" is of great significance in the lives of Pentecostal people, and is felt by them to be the basis of the superiority of their religious belief over that of other religions. They also view "possession" as related to health.

Possession by the Holy Spirit

The Latin-American Assembly of God holds prayer meetings every Friday night. Some of the more devout members of the congregation fast during the day, taking nothing but water, in order to prepare themselves for "receiving the Holy Spirit." One Friday night during the summer of 1955 the service began at 7:30 P.M., with a prayer in Spanish said by a layman of the congregation. Following the opening prayer some hymns were sung in Spanish, many with a lively rhythm. Several members of the congregation kept time to the beat by clapping their hands or tapping their feet. The singing was accompanied by a piano, mandolin, and cornet.

Between the hymns members of the group stood up and gave "testimonials." One of these was given by a man who said that when he was a soldier in the Korean War and was wounded and in an army hospital in Japan, he was not expected to live. However, he said, his faith in God caused the Holy Spirit to come down and possess him, thus saving his life. During the service, members of the congregation expressed their agreement and enthusiasm by shouting "Amen," "Aleluya," or *"Oye, Señor!"* (Hear me, Lord).

After the testimonials, the pastor delivered a sermon. For the first twenty minutes the people listened quietly, then began talking softly, humming, or murmuring "Amen." Shortly after this, an older woman began to be "possessed," wailing in a high-pitched voice, sobbing, and flexing her body back and forth with arms extended over her head. Soon other members of the group were "filled with the Holy Spirit," some speaking rapidly in loud voices, first in Spanish and then in "unknown tongues," the latter thought to be a sign that the speaker was "possessed" and the Holy Ghost was speaking through him. During the remainder of the sermon about one-fourth of the members of the group became "possessed," while others prayed aloud or cried. The service ended with a hymn and a closing prayer.

Faith Healing

Among Mexican-American Protestants, particularly those of Pentecostal sects, there is a great deal of emphasis on the healing power of God through faith and prayer. (The Catholic reliance on prayers, vows, and offerings to saints and Virgins was mentioned previously. Several churches have special organizations whose function is helping the sick to be healed through prayer; one such organization was mentioned above.) There are two sects—neither of them in Mayfair, however—among San Jose Mexican-Americans that openly oppose the use of medicines and the services of physicians. One is a Jehovah's Witnesses sect which has no church in Mayfair but sends missionaries into the area. The second is a Pentecostal sect in a community near Mayfair whose minister is said to be "against doctors" on the theory that resorting to medical care is an admission of insufficient faith in the power of God to heal the sick.

The position of Mayfair Pentecostal ministers on faith healing, however, does not discourage use of medical facilities. One minister explained the position of his church in this way: "We sincerely believe in the healing power of faith and prayer. I know it works, and even the doctors admit it. I usually tell my congregation that medical science, like everything else in the world, is learned by the grace of God. God allowed the science of medicine to be created. Therefore you should pray and have faith in God to heal you. But the evidence of God's healing power is in such things as the X ray for TB, which shows when you are cured. The medical doctor may be the instrument of God, and you should give God a chance to work through his instruments."

In spite of the official position of Mayfair churches on the concept of faith healing, there are individuals in various congregations who believe that certain persons are magically endowed with curative powers. Beatriz, a member of a Pentecostal sect, was a patient at the county tuberculosis sanatorium in 1955. She said, "One of my friends who belongs to the same church I attend gave me a subscription to the *Oral Roberts Healing Magazine*.[5] I read every copy of it. Oral Roberts can really cure people by faith—he can do real miracles. He had a big rally down in Fresno a few years ago, and a lot of Mexican people I know went down to attend it. When he touches them, people who have been paralyzed begin to move and cross-eyed people get their eyes straightened out. He can cure TB, too. He used to have TB himself, but he cured himself by faith, and now

[5] Oral Roberts is a Protestant evangelist and faith healer, not affiliated with any particular church. During 1955, he presented a fifteen-minute television program each Sunday afternoon which was very popular with both Catholic and Protestant Spanish-speaking patients at the county tuberculosis sanatorium.

he is well and can use his lungs better than ever. He can yell real loud when he preaches. If I had the chance, I'd go to Oral Roberts and have him cure me."

PROTESTANT GROUPS AND COMMUNITY LIFE

Pentecostal churches in Mayfair have many religious and social activities for their congregations. Members spend a large part of their leisure time at the church, and their social relationships are generally restricted to friendships with fellow parishioners. One Pentecostal woman reported, "Almost all my friends go to the Apostolic Church. I don't seem to make friends very well with other Protestants or with Catholics. I find that so many of the things that they want to do are sinful, and our church forbids these things. I guess I just don't have much in common with those people."

Members of nonpossessional Protestant churches, however, often establish friendships with those of other religious beliefs; differences in religious affiliation in Mayfair generally do not interfere with social relationships between Catholics, Baptists, Methodists, and non-churchgoers. The Pentecostal sects, on the other hand, form cliques in the community as a result of their social semi-isolation from their neighbors. They tend to constitute a socially distinct group and take little part in community life.

In discussing the role of religious differences in Mexican-American social structure, Broom and Shevky [7] observe that the church is a force for retention of Mexican culture patterns among Mexican-Americans in the United States, and that it deters assimilation of the group into the majority culture. A second point they make is that competition between Catholic and Protestant churches intensifies social cleavages in Mexican-American communities. Both these points are borne out by observation in Mayfair.

6

THE PATTERN OF FAMILY LIFE

MANY FACETS OF Mexican-American life play a part in the recognition and treatment of illness. Previous chapters have suggested that education, economic level, and religious beliefs all affect medical attitudes and practices among the people of east San Jose. None of these, however, exerts a more powerful influence on individual health practices than do the customs which prevail in the homes of Spanish-speaking people. Among Sal si Puedes families there are beliefs and customs regarding pregnancy, childbirth, and infant care which directly influence maternal and child health practices. Customs and beliefs concerning food affect nutrition. The pattern of family authority may determine when an individual is free to seek and receive medical aid. Attitudes toward the aged are involved in determining whether or not an elderly person suffering from serious chronic disease will be hospitalized. The individual's relations to his family and kinship group influence his personal adjustment and mental health. Special consideration is given in this chapter to conflicts between Mexican and American culture patterns in home life and the effects of those conflicts on young people whose lives are shaped by two cultural traditions.

LIFE CYCLE

The following pages contain descriptions of some Sal si Puedes families, the events of the cycle of birth and death in the barrio, relations between family members, and household activities.

CONCEPTION AND PREGNANCY

The people of Sal si Puedes believe that childbearing is both a privilege and an obligation of married women. Generally the people are fond of children and have large families. For example, the 37 married women of the neighborhood forty years of age and over had a total of 203 living children, a mean average of 5.5 children for each mother. Married women who have only one child or no children at all are sympathetically counseled by other women of the community who frequently offer advice and prescriptions for aiding conception. Barrenness is attributed to a variety of causes. Rosa's inability to conceive after the delivery of her first child, for example, was ascribed to her husband's stomach ulcers. Carmen thought that her own inability to have additional children was the fault of a change of dietary habits: "My mother had fifteen children, lived to be a hundred and three years old, and never went to a doctor or a hospital. She had all of her children with a midwife and had no trouble at all with childbirth. But even though I wanted more children, I was able to have just two. I think it's because of the food we have to eat here in California. Everybody is in such a hurry that the women can't cook the food right—we eat it half-raw; no wonder we have trouble!" Carmen was sure that raw food was to blame for her difficulties; she mentioned only parenthetically that she had had an operation (later identified as an hysterectomy) shortly after the birth of her second baby. (For further discussion of diet and beliefs concerning health and disease, see chapter 7.)

Almost every older woman of the barrio has an inventory of the methods thought to aid conception. If home remedies are not effective in aiding conception, a woman may be taken by friends or relatives to see a *curandera*. Some of the home remedies for barrenness and methods used by one of the most popular curanderas in the area are described in the following chapter.

Not all Sal si Puedes women have faith in these remedies; younger women are particularly skeptical. One laughingly remarked, "My mother and all her friends can tell me a dozen things to do to help me get pregnant, but none of them work. The only thing to do if you want more children is pray to God and the Holy Mother to send you another child—then if God wills it, you will have other children." Teresa, who has worked as a practical nurse in several San Jose hospitals, said, "A lot of women ask me what they can do to get pregnant. I don't believe in all these remedies that people use, so I just tell them to go to a doctor and he will find out what the trouble is."

Although most Sal si Puedes families are large, the people of the barrio are divided in their opinions about family size. Parents with only one or two children often feel that they "don't have enough." "It's hard on kids to be alone or have only one brother or sister," Paula remarked. Older parents (about thirty-five years of age and over) generally favor large families. Younger people, however, follow the "Anglo pattern" of desiring fewer children. Ramón, in his early thirties, is the father of three children. "Three is all I want, too," he insisted. "I think the Mexican people have too many kids and that's one reason they can't get ahead."

Theoretical differences between Catholic and Protestant attitudes toward contraception are not reflected in actual family size: Protestant families average as many children as do Catholic families. The attitudes toward birth control which people express verbally, however, seem to be influenced by religious considerations.

A Spanish-speaking doctor in San Jose reported that he has very few requests from Mexican-American women for information about contraception. "I think it may be because they don't like to discuss these things—it embarrasses them, especially with a male doctor. Then, too, most are Catholic, and even though a woman might like to use contraceptives, she would worry about what other people will think of her if she does—they don't want people to think they're going against their religion." Several public health nurses in Spanish-speaking districts reported that they had spoken to Mexican-American mothers about the use of contraceptives to regulate family size, and that many women said, "I'd like to use something to keep from getting pregnant, but my husband wouldn't like it." When the nurses explained that diaphragm-type contraceptives did not interfere with sexual enjoyment, most women insisted that their husbands still wouldn't approve: "They just wouldn't feel right about it."

Expectant mothers try to avoid severe emotional upsets lest the unborn child be affected in some way. When Soledad's husband slapped her and threatened to beat her, her mother rushed her to a curandera for preventive treatment; Soledad was apparently unharmed, but it was feared that her emotional upset might cause the child to contract an illness. Manny, a teen-age boy, reported that he was a twin: "But once when my mother was pregnant, my father got drunk and beat her up; it scared her real bad. Because of that my twin sister was born dead."

Paula asserted that women in California have premature deliveries or miscarriages because there are so many earthquakes. "An earthquake can cause some women who are expecting to get so scared that it causes them to have the babies too soon. A very strong earthquake can cause the baby to get turned around and then be born *con nalgas adelante* [in breech position]." [1]

When Maria was expecting her last baby, she tried to avoid seeing unpleasant sights and becoming emotionally upset. One day she heard a noise in the yard, and a child began to cry. She quickly made the sign of the cross and went to the kitchen door to see what had happened. One of her comadre's children had struck his little sister with his bicycle. When Maria saw that none of her own children was involved in the accident, she said "Thank God," and crossed herself again. The hurt child continued to scream, however, and Maria asked a visitor to go outside and see what was wrong with the little girl. She explained that she could not go herself because she was "afraid for the baby" and feared that she might see an unpleasant sight that would injure or "mark" the child in some way.

[1] Parsons [34] reported the following stories from a Oaxacan village in Mexico: "Be'ta told me of a stillbirth which occurred as the result of the earthquake. She imputed it primarily to the wind of the quake . . . and secondarily to the fright [*espanto*] of the mother. At San Dionisio a faulty presentation, arm first, was imputed also to the earthquake which had misplaced the fetus."

One example of supposed prenatal influence was that of a child born with a large hairy mole, which the mother believed was caused by being frightened by a cat during her pregnancy.

Several older people attributed the cleft palate of a child to a prenatal experience. It was thought that the pregnant mother had been exposed to an eclipse of the moon.[2] A public health nurse reported that she had seen Mexican-American mothers hang keys from their waists to "lock the child in" as protection against eclipses.

A few people expressed the opinion that certain foods can "mark a child" and hence should be avoided by expectant mothers. For example, some do not eat fish for fear the baby will have scales. This common Mexican belief that a child may be "marked" by the mother's prepartum diet [3] is not widespread in east San Jose. Most people had heard the idea expressed, but it was generally dismissed as a superstition.

The majority, however, believes that highly spiced foods eaten by an expectant mother may impair the child's health. Several people claimed that if an expectant mother ate very hot chilies it might cause the child to have poor digestion later in life. At a baby shower the guest of honor asked that her enchiladas be made without chili sauce. Lupe, another guest, explained, "A pregnant woman shouldn't eat very hot foods, such as a lot of hot chilies. If she eats too many of them, the baby, after it is born, is likely to have *chincual*." [4] Chincual is described as a "disease" characterized by redness and sores on the buttocks (evidently a sort of "diaper rash"). Lupe qualified her statement, however, by remarking that some babies are more susceptible to the disease than others: "I ate hot chilies when I was pregnant, but my babies didn't have it. But then my sister ate them too, and both of her babies had chincual real bad." Another young mother of the barrio, Elvira, said, "Some people say that chincual is caused when a woman eats a lot of hot foods while she

---

[2] Parsons [34] reported from the village of Mitla: "During an eclipse of the moon a prospective mother should not venture outdoors lest the child be born with a hairlip or other imperfection or deformity, without ears, for example."

[3] Foster [16] reported from a village in Michoacan that Tarascan Indian parents-to-be "must not eat rabbit for fear the child will have big ears, nor do they eat squirrel for fear it will have big teeth and a long nose."

[4] *Chincual*, given the Spanish spelling in San Jose, is a term derived from the Aztecan *tzin* (rump) and *cualitztli* (decay). Foster [16] reported from Mexico: "If chiles are eaten after the first 3 months [of pregnancy] the child will suffer from *chinkual*, cutaneous eruptions which last for several months after birth."

is pregnant. I don't think that's right, though, because I always ate hot foods while I was carrying all of my kids, and none of them ever had it. I think it's either that the baby's food doesn't agree with it, or because of soap or bleach in the diapers. Some of these soaps that you buy in the stores now are really hard on a baby's skin."

Barrio residents are very reluctant to discuss abortion and abortionists. Most people, when asked about "getting rid of an unwanted child," replied categorically that Mexican people always want their babies and never do this sort of thing. Only one intentional abortion was reported. Juana told the following story: "My sister got married when she was very young—only sixteen—and soon she had two children. After that she got pregnant three or four more times, but she didn't have those babies because her husband started taking her to a place in Mexicali [Mexico] for abortions. Her husband told her that he didn't want all those kids, that he couldn't support them. Finally I got some of my relatives to go with me to talk to my sister about it, and we talked her out of going there any more. We told her that it was dangerous to her health—that she could get an infection and die. Then her kids would be left alone and her husband wouldn't suffer—he'd just get himself another woman. So my sister decided to tell her husband she wouldn't go any more. She had three more kids after that—that's five children in all."

Although it was not possible to collect much concrete information on the incidence of abortion in Mayfair, there is some indication that intentional abortion is infrequent. Involuntary abortion or miscarriage is quite frequent, however, and there are very few women past the childbearing years who have not had one or more miscarriages. The role that emotional upsets and unusual events (earthquakes, accidents) are thought to play in miscarriage is mentioned above. A few miscarriages and stillbirths were attributed to improper medical treatment. Marta reported, "My comadre's daughter was under the care of an American doctor when she was expecting her baby. One night she got real sick, and it looked like she was going to have the baby right then, even though it wasn't her time yet. So I called that doctor on the phone and told him about it, but he just said I must be crazy, that she wasn't due for another three months. But she got worse, and we kept calling that doctor back on the telephone. Finally, a long time after that, he came out to see my comadre's daughter, and when he did come he took one look at her and said, 'Call an ambulance.' When they got her to the hospital, she had a miscarriage. So she spent all her money and still lost her baby." Marta felt that the doctor was definitely at fault: "I don't know why that doctor wouldn't believe us when we said he should come quick. Maybe he was just lazy, or maybe he didn't think we knew anything—that we were stupid."

Women prefer to remain in the privacy of their homes during the last month or two before delivery because of the "embarrassment" of being seen in public in the late stages of pregnancy. Marta, in her eighth month of pregnancy, said that she had stopped going to public gatherings: "I don't think I'll go to church any more until after the baby is born. The last time I went, Father stopped right in the middle of the rosary and told me I'd better sit down. I was so ashamed I could have died!"

Most parents want children of both sexes. Men show a slight preference for sons and women for daughters. Parents who have older children of both sexes generally have no preferences as to the sex of a new baby. Irene, expecting her ninth child, said, "By this time, I don't really care which it is—a boy or a girl, what's the difference?"

There are many factors involved in whether or not a woman will go to a doctor for prenatal care. These will be discussed in the following chapter.

BIRTH AND POSTNATAL CARE

Most deliveries are in hospitals, but occasionally a mother has her baby at home. Young women generally consider the county hospital a good place to have babies. Paula said, "My sister had fourteen babies there, and I guess it must be a pretty good place because all of them were healthy and my sister still has a figure like a young girl." Older women and a minority of young mothers dislike hospital deliveries because American obstetrical procedures differ so much from traditional Mexican childbirth practices.

Manuela said it was too bad that *parteras* (midwives) were not allowed to deliver babies in California: "In Mexico—and in Arizona and New Mexico and Texas, too—most of the women have their babies with the partera. All the women I know from those places liked the parteras much better than a regular medical doctor. The parteras seem to take more interest in them, come to their homes and stay with the mother from the time the labor pains begin. They do other things, too—massage them, rub them with oil to relax them, and give them hot teas to drink, like *orégano* or *manzanilla* [camomile] tea." A well-to-do Mexican-American family who lived in another part of San Jose were said to have imported a licensed Mexican-American midwife from Texas to attend the mother. Sal si Puedes families, however, cannot afford such an expense, and there are no licensed practicing midwives among the San Jose Spanish-speaking people.

Doña Serafina, a long-time resident of Sal si Puedes, was once a midwife in Mexico before she came to the United States. Although she is not licensed to deliver children under California law, many expectant mothers of the neighborhood go to her for advice during their pregnancies. Doña Serafina is now eighty years of age, however, and is able to do nothing more than give advice.

Concepción, who has given birth to fifteen children, told of her experiences during the births of some of her children: "I had my first baby in Mexico, and my husband and mother helped me to have the baby. Just a little while after that, we moved to California and got a house in Milpitas [near San Jose]. We were strangers here then, and when the time came for me to have my next child we didn't know where to turn. Finally we decided to bring an Italian midwife [licensed] from Santa Clara. This woman was no good, though—she did almost nothing, even though the baby was upside down [breech presentation]. She should have turned the baby around, at least. When I began to have my pains, I saw that the partera was going to do nothing, and I thought, 'Why doesn't this woman massage me? Where are the oils for rubbing?' Then, after the birth, she didn't even bind my abdomen."

After this unpleasant experience with a midwife, Concepción and her family decided that it would be best if she had her next baby at the hospital in San Jose. "This was terrible, too," she asserted. "As soon as my pains started, I went to the hospital. But they did nothing to help me have the baby, and I lay there for three days before the baby was born. I was in a ward with fourteen other women, all of them yelling and screaming, and they wouldn't let me see my husband. I got so nervous that I thought I couldn't stand it any longer."

Concepción, who speaks only Spanish, felt that she was badly neglected at the Anglo hospital. She was isolated from her husband

and other relatives, given no personal antepartum care, and, because of her language problem, did not know what she could expect of the hospital staff or what was expected of her. Placed in a large ward, she was embarrassed by having to undergo labor in a room full of strange women. Her clothes were taken away, and she was left clad in only a hospital gown, which she considered insufficient covering. When, in desperation, she wrapped herself in a towel to go in search of her husband and other relatives, a nurse, unable to communicate with Concepción verbally, tried to get her back in bed by means of physical force. Concepción was confused, frightened, and angry with the whole hospital situation. She was delighted when the baby was born on the hospital cart in transit to the delivery room; she thought this was a very good joke on the whole system. When the time came for Concepción to have her next child, she "waited too long" to go to the hospital and was delivered at home, assisted by her mother and younger sister.

The story of Concepción's first hospital delivery is not typical of the experiences of Mexican-American mothers in the community, but neither is it unique. Concepción was newly arrived from Mexico at the time, whereas most of her neighbors are either American born or have lived in the United States for several years. Although many would prefer to be delivered at home, there is general acceptance of obstetrical services provided by the local county hospital.

Almost all mothers, even those who are young and American born, regard the postpartum weeks as a critical period. A new mother should be very careful during *la cuarentena,* the forty days after delivery, to observe certain dietary restrictions and follow certain procedures which are thought to restore her to normal health. The most common criticism made in Sal si Puedes of hospital maternity care is that no provision is made for carrying out the postpartum procedures which Mexican-Americans consider essential. Rosa, an American-born woman who is considered quite rash by most of her associates because she has adopted so many Anglo customs, described an experience she had after the delivery of her first child: "Most of us think that it's very important during the first forty days for a new mother to bind her abdomen with a tight binder. We usually make them out of unbleached muslin or some other strong material. Most people think that this helps all of these organs in the stomach to go back where they belong, and especially to push the hips together. When I had my baby, I remember that I was really upset when the nurse came in on the third day after my delivery, took off the binder, and left it off. I asked the nurse if she wasn't going to put it back on, or if she wanted me to have my husband or some of my friends bring my binder from home so that I could wear it when I was discharged from the hospital. The nurse told me that I wasn't supposed to be wearing it any more and that I must leave it off. Well, I did what she said, but I was sure worried about it because I was afraid it was going to leave my stomach flabby and make me get real fat."

Almost all mothers are firm in their belief that certain foods should be avoided during the postpartum period, lest the health of either the mother or the nursing infant be affected. Foods which should be avoided are: hot chilies, pickles, vinegar (or any food prepared with vinegar), tomatoes, spinach, pork of all kinds (including bacon), and most fruits. Fruits thought to be especially harmful are bananas, grapefruit, and other citrus fruits. These fruits are thought to be "too acid" and cause varicose veins in mothers who eat them during this period. Some vegetables (e.g., spinach) are bad because they are "too cold for the stomach." (For a discussion of "hot" and "cold" foods, see chapter 7.) Opinion in the barrio is divided about the wisdom of including beans in the postpartum diet. Some mothers say beans can be eaten if they are prepared without hot chilies, but others insist that they should be eaten sparingly by nursing mothers because "too many are bad for the baby's stomach."

The ideal postpartum diet consists of foods which are thought to assure adequate lactation and rich milk. Some of these are: chicken, either fried or in soup; tortillas toasted crisp; eggs; toasted bread; milk; cooked cereals, as oatmeal, rice, or *atole* (a thin gruel of corn or other cereal prepared with milk and chocolate); chocolate; and *panes dulces* (Mexican sweet yeast rolls). Meats other than pork may be eaten, but only chicken is regarded as particularly beneficial.

A Mexican custom of taking gifts of food to a new mother is observed by a few people recently arrived from Mexico. Favorite dishes to be given are chicken soup and toasted tortillas. Most American-born residents, however, do not observe this tradition.

Many mothers observe dietary restrictions not only for the forty days after delivery but limit their choice of foods until the child is weaned. A small group of young mothers who consider themselves "modern" begin eating other foods after three or four weeks.

Rubbing the back with a mixture of warm olive oil (or melted lard) and powdered sulphur is thought to be good for keeping a new mother's lungs and chest clear, thereby assuring healthy breasts and a quantity of rich milk. To end lactation when a child is weaned mothers bind the breasts and apply camphorated oil as a massage.

Sal si Puedes women generally regard pregnancy and childbirth as trying, but not altogether unpleasant. There are many restrictions in diet which most regard as very important; the avoidance of prohibited foods can become tedious, particularly when they are staple items of Mexican-American diet (tomatoes, pork, chilies). But the discomforts of pregnancy, childbirth, and rigid diet are counterbalanced by the special care and consideration afforded expectant and new mothers by friends and relatives. Particular care is taken that a woman in confinement shall not be exposed to unpleasant or upsetting experiences. Friends, neighbors, and relatives come to visit, help with housework and child care, bring gifts, and offer personal attention and social support. Strong bonds of kinship and friendship protect and comfort young women during this life crisis.

INFANCY

Although about 40 per cent of all infants born to Sal si Puedes families are breast fed, by three months after birth only about 20 per cent are still being nursed. Those who are changed from breast feeding to formula are generally weaned from the breast at about six to eight weeks of age. At this time the baby can be bottle fed in its bed, and busy mothers feel that it is much easier to prepare a bottle than to take time to nurse the child.

Many mothers believe that nursing prevents conception, and some women continue breast feeding as a contraceptive measure. If a woman who is nursing a child does conceive, the infant is weaned immediately and put on a formula. Most older women believe that bottle feeding is "unnatural" and will inevitably lead to the child's falling ill. They think that a baby should be nursed for three years. One young mother explained, "I know the older people say to let a child nurse for a long time—some say three or four years —but most of us wean our babies when they are twelve to eighteen months old or younger. But there is one thing that most mothers do believe: They don't like to use a feeding schedule because they think a baby should be fed whenever it cries or is fretful. Whenever the baby is hungry, a mother likes to feed it."

One mother of six children commented, "Most of the women I know believe that a bottle-fed baby will suffer from stomach trouble later in life. Mothers will usually nurse their babies if there's any way to do it. I nursed my first four children, but I guess I got lazy with the last two because I put them right on formulas when they were born. I think I'm getting too old for it now, and I don't like to be tied down to a nursing schedule. But my sister is always telling me that the last two will have weak stomachs when they get older. Maybe she's right, but I think the most important thing is letting the baby get used to one way of eating and then sticking to that. I don't think it matters if you nurse them or give them a formula, or whether you feed them at regular times or just when they're hungry—the important thing is to do it the same way all the time. If you put a baby on a schedule when it's born, you have to keep it that way. And you shouldn't change a baby to a schedule from eating when it cries, or it will get sick."

Generally, infants are fed only milk until they are about three or four months old, at which time mothers usually begin to add a little cooked cereal to the diet. Favorite cereals are oatmeal and creamed wheat. Most infants begin getting a little fruit when they are about six months old; bananas are given sparingly, however, because of the belief that a child who is fed bananas, particularly a small infant, may suffer from *empacho*, a stomach disorder. (For discussion of empacho and other folk-disease concepts, see chapter 7.)

Although infants may be given a little solid food during the first year of life, the quantity is usually small as long as the child is nursing or receiving formula. The use of vitamins varies a great deal from one mother to the next. For example, a few are meticulous in giving their infants cod-liver oil, some give none at all, and most give it at irregular intervals.

Recently, obesity among infants and small children in the barrio has become a problem. There is a current fad of giving sweetened, high-calorie milk to infants. Teresa reported, "Not long ago I took the baby [a girl of about fourteen months] to the doctor for a check-up. The doctor told me that the baby's too fat, and that she weighs just twice what is normal for her age. He told me to put her on skimmed milk and cut out sweet fruits from her food. Well, I'll tell you, I'm not going to put that baby on a diet because she is healthy and happy just the way she is!" During the conversation Teresa, who had given the child breakfast earlier in the day, fed her child a mid-morning snack consisting of a cup of whole milk flavored with coffee and table sugar (two teaspoons), a bakery doughnut, and about half of a pan dulce, a large breakfast roll. Teresa seemed to take pride in having a fat baby and was annoyed with the doctor for having suggested that overfeeding of infants constituted a health problem.

Public health nurses in Santa Clara County who visit migrant Spanish-speaking families report that some infants are swaddled. This was not noted in Sal si Puedes except when a very small infant was to be taken outside the house. The procedure was a simple one: the baby was simply rolled, "mummy" fashion, from just below the armpits to the feet in a cotton receiving blanket before being bundled up for the excursion.

Infants' fingernails are not cut very early. Some parents believe that if this is done before the baby is six weeks old, it will make the child weak. Mothers who do not trim their babies' nails may dress them in mittens to prevent their scratching themselves.

As Foster [16] reports, in parts of Mexico the "hair of young children is not cut until they are able to talk," because it "retards the learning process." This belief about allowing a child's hair to grow is not held by Sal si Puedes mothers. One said, "Some of the old people think a girl's hair shouldn't be cut, but nobody pays any attention to that now; they keep their little girls' hair cut short."

Circumcision of male infants is considered a procedure of dubious value. One mother explained that she didn't have her baby circumcised "because it's unnatural and makes the baby look so ugly." A district nurse commented that it is unusual to find a Mexican baby circumcised: "Most mothers prefer not to have the operation done. I'm not sure why, but I think it has something to do with the concept of modesty." Mercedes said, "None of our people had their boys circumcised in the old days, but some modern mothers have it done now. The old people think it's terrible and tell the young mothers they are breaking God's law. The old people say it's unnatural and that's one reason the babies get sick."

Mexican-American infants are held and fondled frequently. Homes are usually full of visitors, and even if a busy mother does not have time to hold an infant, a visiting aunt, grandmother, or neighbor may hold the child. When infants fret and begin to cry, they are generally fed or given pacifiers. If feeding does not stop an infant's crying, the mother usually holds the child, petting or rocking it in her arms or bouncing it on her knee or on her shoulder. Older infants are given various things to play with—sometimes a toy, but just as frequently a comb, a compact, a cigarette case, or a key ring. Most mothers are careful to keep the infant's genitalia covered when diapering the child, placing a fresh diaper over the genital area before removing the soiled one. Subsequent cleaning is done underneath the fresh diaper, the mother peeking under one edge of the cloth.

Infant clothing is much the same as that used by Anglo parents, except that most mothers pin small religious medals to their babies' dresses. Female infants generally have their ears pierced by the mother or a female relative or friend when the child is about two months of age, and small gold earrings are placed in the ears.

Among Catholic families, baptism is the most important ceremonial event during infancy. Rosa described baptismal procedure: "In the old days in Mexico, when a child was born the friends of the parents used to come to the house within the first few days after the delivery and ask for the baby [that is, ask to be the child's godparents] for baptism. The first ones to ask were the godparents, and those who came late would just have to wait until another baby was born if they wanted to be the padrinos [godparents]. Now here in San Jose the parents usually have someone in mind to be the padrinos before the baby is born, and they ask these friends to baptize the baby."

If a child is born alive, but dies shortly after birth, it is sometimes taken to the church to be baptized before burial, but more often, some friends will be asked to go to the hospital with some holy water and perform a lay baptism. A stillborn child is not baptized, but is buried without any ceremony. Other aspects of the godparent relationship are discussed below in the topic on compadrazgo.

Age of children at baptism varies considerably. A few are baptized within a few weeks after birth, but some are two or three years old. Average age of infants at christening is about six to eight months.

CHILDHOOD

Children are generally considered to be past infancy when a younger sibling is born. When a child learns to walk and talk fairly well, he is allowed to play about the house without much parental supervision. Children two and three years of age are allowed to play outside in their own or a neighbor's yard, but are usually watched (sometimes not too closely) by an older brother or sister. Children four or older are left to amuse themselves however they can in house or yard, playing with neighbor children their own age or taken in tow by older siblings.

Small children have a few toys, but they show less interest in them than Anglo children of the same age. This may be because there are usually other children nearby to play with or observe. Small children seem to enjoy being with adults, listening to conversation and observing adult activities, as much as playing with toys. Parents do not seem to be "bothered" by having children around; they are seldom sent to another part of the house or outside unless they are particularly noisy and rowdy.

Parents talk very little to their small children except to answer questions or give instructions. Mothers often talk to each other about children who are present, however. When a young child is being talked about in his presence, he usually lowers his head, hides his face behind his mother's skirt, or hides bodily behind a piece of furniture. Children from one to three years old cry frequently, but children four and older rarely cry unless they are hurt or frightened.

Barrio parents are aware of sibling jealousy; it is considered a usual thing for a second-youngest child to be resentful of a new baby. Jealous children are generally teased or ignored when showing signs of resentment of a younger child. A small child may be punished, however, for physically harming an infant.

The most widely used means of control of children is fear. Threats of physical punishment are common both from parents and from older siblings. Ismael commented, "I can't understand parents who let their kids run wild and don't make them behave. Some people let their children interrupt adults when they are talking, hang on to their mother, and show no respect for their elders. Sometimes you have to spank a child to make him respect you. Once when my oldest boy was just a baby, he got started crying and wouldn't stop. Finally I got a little switch and told him that he'd better shut up or he was going to get switched. He stopped crying right away and he hasn't cried like that any more."

When Sara's two younger children, ages three and four, are annoy-ing her when she is busy with her housework, she usually ignores them for a while or tells them quietly to leave her alone and let her do her work. If the children continue to vex her, she is likely first to shout, "Shut up!" Later she may threaten to hit them with a belt, and finally she may call an older brother or sister to take them into another part of the house. If Sara's patience is exhausted, she may instruct the older child to hit them or, as a last resort, spank them herself.

Older children are punished less often, but their punishment may be severe. Physical punishment of older children is usually left to an older brother or to the father, although a mother may slap a child, particularly a daughter. Younger brothers are sometimes beaten rather severely by older ones. These beatings are not rebuked by adults—in fact, the older child is often instructed to administer the blows. Young children are usually quite as much in awe of an older brother as they are of their parents.

Some parents complain that their children do not receive rigid enough discipline at school and claim that teachers are much too lax in their treatment of students. Paula said, "I used to get real mad at Tony's teacher because she wouldn't make him behave at school. I would always tell the teacher to go ahead and whip him if he is a bad boy—but the teacher doesn't like to do it, so the kids run all over her. They get used to doing whatever they please, and we can't do anything with them at home."

Young children are sometimes punished by isolating them in an unoccupied room of the house (as the bathroom) or by keeping them indoors when they want to play outside.

One mother was observed trying to control her four-year-old son by exploiting fear of doctors and hypodermic injections. She once threatened the child with a "shot" in the presence of a public health nurse. The nurse gently reminded the mother that "we like to have children come to the doctor sometimes when they don't need a shot." The nurse then asked the little boy if he would like to come to the child-health conference sometime and watch the doctor examine his new baby sister. The child was already afraid, however, and without hesitation said "No!"

Children are encouraged to develop independence at an early age. Even a very young child who clings to his mother or father is considered to be "spoiled." Ramón remarked that his two-year-old son, who kept clinging to his father's leg, "is sure spoiled—I've really got him spoiled." This took place at about eight or nine o'clock at night, and the child seemed quite sleepy. Ramón finally picked up the boy and kissed him, but only after apologizing to those present for his child's behavior.

On one occasion Paula was sitting in the living room of a neighbor's house talking to several of her friends. Her eight-year-old boy came up beside her and kissed her on the cheek. She turned to him and said, "Don't do that!" and pushed him away. The child withdrew a step or two and asked, "Don't you love me any more?" Paula smiled a little, but said, in a gruff voice, "No!" The boy shrugged his shoulders and walked into the other room. Paula turned to her comadre and remarked, "I don't know what's wrong with him—he's always trying to kiss me. He thinks that just because his father plays with him sometimes, that he can play with me."

Most children get fairly consistent training in working independently. Three-year-old Rudy and his mother were visiting his aunt one day. Rudy asked his aunt for an apple, and she told him to get one from the kitchen. Before he had a chance to eat it, however, he dropped it on the floor and it rolled under the bed. He went to his mother and told her that he wanted his apple, and she told him to get it himself. At first he was unsuccessful, but no one made a move to help him. After ten minutes of struggle, Rudy finally succeeded in recovering his apple, joyfully picked it up, wiped it on his trousers, and began to nibble.

On another occasion a man was loading some household goods into a truck. When he had finished loading it, two boys about ten and twelve years of age got a rope and attempted to lash the load to the truckbed. The man interfered only to tell the boys (not show them) how to tie the rope more effectively and to make sure the knots were secure. Parents generally do not interfere with the completion of a job assigned to a child. Men do not take tools away from their sons or push them out of the way to finish the job themselves.

Adults seldom give detailed instructions or stand over a child to supervise his work.

Parents are not always consistent about training their children to be independent, however. Paula's behavior toward the same child that she pushed away was, on another occasion, quite different. One night Paula's son had overheard his parents and some of their friends discussing a series of episodes involving ghosts, death, omens, mountain lions, and other things which might seem frightening to a child. Paula reported: "Tony [the child] woke up during the night having bad dreams. He couldn't go back to sleep and was up pacing the floor in his room at two in the morning. I wanted to go see what was wrong with him, but his father said, 'Leave him alone and let him be a man.' At first I did what my husband said, but then he got mad when Tony's walking around kept him awake—he got up and locked Tony in his room. Then I got really mad; I got up and went in and slept with Tony in his bed all the rest of the night."

Parents sometimes use fear to regulate their children's diets. Teresa's three-year-old boy, who was always begging for a cup of coffee, was told that if he drank coffee he would grow horns. Rosa reported that she used to tell her daughter the same thing, but the child used to worry about it: "Every time I'd give her a spoonful of coffee in her milk, I'd notice her feeling her forehead afterwards to see if the horns had sprouted yet."

Boys and girls play together until they are seven or eight years old, but at about that time they are encouraged to play separately. Children nine to eleven years old are influential in encouraging younger children to restrict their associations to members of their own sex. Eleven-year-old Betty reported that she did not like to walk to school with her nine-year-old brother: "I feel ashamed because he walks with me and tries to make up to my girl friends. I tell him to walk with the other boys."

Parents avoid sexual discussions with preadolescent children except for giving them general instructions to "stay away from boys," or "leave the girls alone." An eleven-year-old girl said, "Last year I had a best girl friend, but my mother didn't like her. That girl went in the dark with the boys and took me with her. My mother doesn't want me to go around with her any more."

Beatriz, a Mexican-born woman of about forty-five, remarked that an American custom which she finds hard to accept is sex education in the schools. "Last week my nephew's little girl, nine years old, came home after seeing a movie at Mayfair School and started asking a lot of questions about menstruation and childbirth. The movie had been all about these things, but the child was too young to understand it. It's a shame to show a movie like that to little children. The little girl's mother had to sit down with her and explain everything long before it was proper. If she had been thirteen or fourteen years old, it would have been all right, but nine is too young for children to be exposed to things like that."

Sal si Puedes children attend school four or five hours daily, depending on their grade. There is no parochial school in east San Jose, and Catholic as well as Protestant children go to public schools.

Children are given regular work to do in most families. Girls of all ages and boys under the age of twelve are expected to help their mothers with housework and care of younger children. Those who are old enough to help with these tasks are kept at home from school to help their mothers an average of one or two days monthly.

Typical chores of girls are: dish washing, sweeping, washing and ironing, preparing "between-meal" snacks for brothers and sisters, dusting or polishing furniture, helping prepare fruit for home canning, and scrubbing shelves, cabinets, and woodwork.

Boys run errands (usually riding their bicycles), burn trash, pull weeds and work in the yard, help their fathers clean the family car, feed domestic animals (chickens, rabbits), clean animal pens, and mend broken household objects.

During the summer months children of both sexes are often expected to accompany one or both of their parents to work in fields or orchards. They may pick berries, prunes, or beans. Some help their mothers cut apricots for drying during the July apricot harvest. Boys or girls may be dispatched to the home of a grandparent, uncle, or aunt to help with extra work.

Children's play does not differ greatly from that of English-speaking children in Mayfair. The main differences are that Sal si Puedes children seldom read for pleasure and there is very little interest in arts or crafts. None was observed coloring with crayons or water colors, modeling with clay, making model cars or airplanes, or making doll clothes. Play is generally social rather than individual. Group games are much more popular than playing with toys.

Little girls' play is frequently in imitation of adult female activities—they "cook" meals of sand or mud, play "house," or dress up in their mothers' cast-off clothing. Other favorite female pastimes are hopscotch, jumping rope, and roller skating. Girls' play is generally less elaborate than that of boys, perhaps because girls have less leisure time after their household chores are finished.

Bicycle riding is a favorite for boys. They also play baseball and touch or tackle football. Most small boys have slingshots at one time or another; they are simply forked sticks equipped with rubber bands for propelling stones. Some boys hide or break their slingshots from time to time, explaining that they are afraid "the police" will catch them (this happens most often when a window has been broken somewhere in the neighborhood).

The presence of a stray cow one afternoon in 1955 led to a pseudo-bullfight. Four or five little boys (aged from seven to ten) saw the cow escape from a nearby pasture and chased her across a vacant lot and into the barrio streets. Another group of slightly older boys on bicycles began chasing the cow and succeeded in herding it into a neighborhood woman's flower garden. The lady of the house came running outside when she saw the cow grazing in her flower beds, and chased the animal away while the boys continued to circle around on their bicycles, laughing and apparently enjoying the show. By this time six or eight other boys and girls had gathered in the street. One of the newcomers had a large piece of red cloth which he brandished about as if it were a *torero's* cape, shouting, *"Toro, toro, aqui!* [Bull, bull, here!]* "* The boys riding bicycles served as impromptu "picadors" and steered the cow in the general direction of the "matador," while the girls clapped their hands and jumped up and down with excitement. Finally two teen-age boys brought the "bullfight" to a close by shooting the cow with a BB-gun. The "bull" galloped away and the show was over.

ADOLESCENCE

Sal si Puedes people make a social distinction between "children" and "teenagers" (or adolescents). Boys are considered adolescents at thirteen or fourteen years of age and girls at twelve to thirteen. Adolescence ends for boys, according to barrio people, when they are eighteen or nineteen years old or when they marry or become self-supporting. Girls are thought "grown up" when they marry or get a "steady job" and are no longer dependent on their parents for support.

With the beginning of adolescence, girls usually begin wearing lipstick and jewelry. Boys, too, begin imitating their older peers; they learn to dance, learn to drive an automobile, and take more interest in their dress and grooming. Both boys and girls begin to take a lively interest in the opposite sex. Boys of thirteen or fourteen form more intense loyalties to neighborhood or street groups and may form gangs.

Adolescents are under parental control to some extent, usually in the form of constant advice and instructions from parents. Many boys and girls of fifteen to eighteen want to drop out of school but may for various reasons remain in attendance (see chap. 3). One reason is that the father may be absent from the home and the mother receives support from the state; in order for her to receive an allowance for a child under eighteen years of age, the child must be in school. The amount of control exercised over adolescents depends on whether the parents are receiving public assistance, whether only one or both parents are in the home, and whether or not there are older brothers in the family. There is more control if the father or an older brother lives in the home. Other relatives and school authorities have some disciplinary influence, but the most effective control of teenagers comes from age mates.

Activities of Teen-age Girls

Barrio adults seem to expect teenagers to do as much work as grown women; school work and household chores leave little free time for girls during the school year. At puberty, girls may be given a little information about menses by their mothers, but rarely receive parental instruction about sexual behavior and conception. Girls of thirteen to fifteen sometimes discuss sexual behavior with each other, but generally their only sources of information on this topic are copies of *True Confessions* and *Modern Romances*, magazines which are secretly passed around among friends and read in private. A crisis arose for one girl when her little brother discovered that she had been hiding such "pornographic" literature under her mattress and threatened to inform her parents of the fact unless she paid him for keeping her secret.

Recreation for older girls consists of visiting with other girls, going to movies, watching television programs, planning and attending parties (usually for both boys and girls, and sometimes including dancing), and going for automobile rides. Many girls are not permitted by their parents to make dates with boys. The girls themselves usually resent this restriction and meet boys without their parents' knowledge. Some openly defy parental authority and follow the Anglo custom of dating. Some parents, particularly those born in Mexico, believe that young girls should be carefully supervised. Beatriz, who has two teen-age daughters, said: "it's hard to know which is best, the Mexican ideas or the American ideas, about letting young girls go out alone at night. My daughters are always telling me I'm old fashioned because I don't like for them to go out alone with young men. I guess times are changing, but I can't get used to it. In Mexico, when I was a young girl, we were never allowed outside after dark without a chaperon. In those days girls were respectable and acted like ladies."

Some girls are content to meet and talk with boys at parties and public gatherings. Cora, aged seventeen, reported: "My parents don't allow me to go out on dates. I used to get very mad and upset about it, but now I've decided it's all right. I didn't like the idea until a couple of years ago when my brother got a girl pregnant and had to marry her. I sure would hate for that to happen to me!"

Sal si Puedes girls are not a "delinquency problem." If there is premarital sex, it is usually with only one partner and rarely leads to promiscuity or other social difficulties. Illegitimacy is usually avoided by hastily arranging a marriage soon after pregnancy is discovered. If for some reason marriage is not possible, the girl's parents or another relative may adopt the child and rear it as their own. In any event the child is accepted as a part of the family, and its birth is not considered much of a social catastrophe. Social workers assert that there is considerably less prostitution among Mexican-American girls in the area than among Anglos. These counselors do believe that there are many "pick-ups" but no formal prostitution.

A few Mexican-American families in San Jose have a formal debut and ball, the *Baile de Quince*, for their daughters on their fifteenth birthdays. Announcement of a girl's presentation party is sometimes made on one of the local Spanish-language radio programs. The debut is usually an expensive undertaking, and none of the families of Sal si Puedes had the ceremony for their daughters during the course of this study. One mother discussed having the party for her daughter, but finally decided that the family could not afford the expense.

Adolescence spans a relatively short period of time for most girls, since fifteen is thought to be a marriageable age, and most girls in the community do actually marry between the ages of sixteen and nineteen.

Activities of Teen-age Boys

When a girl reaches adolescence, her activities are fairly well defined for her by her social group. It is expected that she will get as much schooling as is convenient, and under her mother's tutelage will acquire the knowledge and skills she will need as a housewife and mother. There is no such clear-cut definition of the behavior expected of teen-age boys.

Boys of fourteen or fifteen do very little work at home; housework is considered appropriate for women and children, but fathers generally do not want their older sons assigned such "feminine" tasks. Boys, like their sisters, are expected to attend school until they are old enough to secure steady employment, but little is demanded of them in the way of daily chores. They are expected to work and earn money during the summer months, but during the school year they are left with a good deal of leisure time, particularly on week ends. This time is usually spent in loafing and conversing with boys their own age.

Burma [8] has pointed out that

In Mexico, it is perfectly normal for men to idle on the street corner; they actually are getting the day's news. . . . In this country that pattern may continue, and the boys may follow their fathers' pattern of loafing and conversing on the streets; they, however, are likely to get into trouble, which did not happen to their fathers. Moreover, in Mexico, the pattern is to release the boy from controls when he is sixteen, so that he may become a man; this means sex, alcohol, and possibly some violence. In the old country it was assumed the boy would have his fling, get it out of his system, and settle down. Here he is considered a delinquent . . . despite his parents' protests that he is not a bad boy.

In San Jose in 1955, local newspapers published a series of articles dealing with a supposed outbreak of delinquency on the part of gangs of Mexican-American youths, so-called "jacket clubs" (thus named because members wear identical jackets with insignia painted or stencilled on the backs). Careful reading of newspaper stories made it clear that what Anglo observers objected to was the mere existence of organized groups of Spanish-speaking boys, and not any specific behavior on their part, since no criminal acts were reported.[5]

There is only one "Jacket club" among Spanish-speaking boys in Mayfair; they call themselves "The Blue Velvets." This group started in 1953 in San Antonio barrio as a street-corner gang who rode around on bicycles. They were then boys of thirteen and fourteen. Now they have bought jackets, have given themselves a name, and are still not delinquent as a group.

In Sal si Puedes there was no organized boys' gang in 1955, although there was an incipient group who "hung around" the corner of the Jackson Avenue Market. These youngsters were fourteen to sixteen years of age, stayed to themselves most of the time, and did not cause trouble as a group. The individual boys who had come to the attention of juvenile authorities had gotten into trouble through chronic truancy for the most part.

There is a general fear among both Spanish-speaking and English-speaking residents of Mayfair that the groups of boys now in the community or some new gang may go further than fighting among themselves and petty delinquency to become a real gang of hoodlums. It is known that there are groups in other parts of San Jose who have been arrested for serious crimes (assault, burglary, automobile theft). Many barrio people express the hope that the juvenile

[5] One of the newspaper articles cited appeared in the *San Jose News*, November 2, 1955: "Three solutions to what may be done to solve the problem of the increasing number of juvenile gangs were outlined this morning at a meeting in the County School Department office, including a 'get tough' proposal. . . . While two other speakers favored organizing such clubs as hot rod organizations and drag races, and working with the Spanish-speaking youths of the area . . . [one participant] . . . said he feels law enforcement is the answer. 'A tough 15-year-old is no different to me than a tough 50-year-old,' . . . [he] . . . said. He further said that if law enforcement officers will make the juvenile trouble-makers realize who's boss, the situation can be solved . . .. [A member] . . . of the County Juvenile Probation Department, said . . . 'The reason these youngsters form gangs is because they don't feel they are a part of the community' . . . He said it is up to the community to work with people who understand the problems of these youngsters, and to find something for them to do . . . another speaker said 90 per cent of the problem could be solved with the organization of drag strips, because most of these 'jacket clubs,' as the gangs are called, are made up of youngsters 'crazy about machinery.' "

authorities will "get tough on these kids and really scare them so they'll know who's boss." One juvenile officer said that "the current juvenile gang scare is due to two things: First, a lot of the boys worked during the summer and saved enough money to buy leather jackets which they decorated with gang insignia. There are a lot of naïve people who confuse clothes with behavior and think if kids dress a certain way, they are hoodlums. Second, there is actually a seasonal increase of petty crime during the winter months because the boys aren't working. The ones who are in school don't usually cause trouble, but there are a good many who have quit school and are too young and unskilled to get work. So they just hang around all winter and get into mischief. Either keeping the boys in school longer or giving them job training would largely solve the Mexican-American delinquency problem. This is borne out by the fact that juvenile crimes practically disappear among Spanish-speaking boys during the summer months when they are all working in the harvest."

A nineteen-year-old boy who had lived in San Jose for a number of years said, "A lot of the trouble the Mexican boys get into is just because they are rebelling against their parents. Mexican parents can't accept American customs and don't approve of their kids' ways. But then the Americans don't ever really accept Mexican kids, either —so the boys have to stick together. That's why the gangs are so important. Some guys really get bitter about this and they carry things so far that they are out to 'get even' with everybody." (For more detailed discussion of delinquency among Mexican-American youths, see Bogardus [5], Harvey [25], Burma [8].)

Another young man, now married and with children of his own, expressed the opinion that boys' gangs are really nothing to worry about: "When I was younger there were about ten or twelve boys that used to wander around at night and get into fights and make a lot of noise. But later on they all got married, and it was real peaceful for a few years. Now the younger boys in those same families are starting up again. Boys get to be teenagers, have parties, fight, get drunk, and make a lot of noise. Then they get married and settle down. It's always the same."

MARRIAGE

Most marriages are arranged by mutual consent of the couple; they simply decide when they want to marry and how long the engagement period will be. In perhaps one marriage out of a hundred, wedding arrangements are made by the parents of the couple. "This is done only in very old-fashioned families," one person observed.

Marriage by elopement occurs from time to time, but an elopement always causes a considerable amount of comment and gossip among people in the community. Of course if either the girl or her fiancé are under legal age and if the parents of either of them object to the match, the parents can appeal to law officers to stop the marriage. However, parents seldom try to stop an elopement by force.

Most engagements are less than three months long, and frequently the wedding is held almost immediately after the announcement of the betrothal. Bridal showers are frequently given during the engagement period, but may follow the wedding.

Most girls marry between the ages of sixteen and nineteen. Men are usually in their early twenties when they marry. In a sample of 40 married couples in the barrio, 34 husbands were older than their wives by an average of 5.4 years, 4 wives were a year or two older than their husbands, and the spouses of 2 couples were the same age.

The basis of marriage is usually mutual affection, but a number of weddings are arranged for other reasons. Premarital pregnancy may result in marriage. If the father of the child is free to marry the mother, he ordinarily does not try to avoid the match. Some men of the community believe that if a young man refuses to marry his girl friend under these circumstances, he can be put in jail.

Single people in their late twenties or thirties may marry because of their age. They feel that it is time they chose a spouse before they get any older, and so a marriage is arranged. Alicia, for example, was thirty-one when she married Esteban. "Everybody thought I was an old maid," she related. "I finally decided I'd better get married before it was too late, so when Esteban asked me to marry him I said yes. Then when I realized what I'd done, I was sad and scared because I wasn't in love or anything else. I was really sorry I had agreed to get married. Before the wedding I cried and cried, but I was too ashamed to back out. But everything is all right now." It is clear to those who know Alicia and Esteban that their relationship certainly is "all right now"; they are one of the most devoted couples in the barrio.

Some girls ascribed their marriages to a desire to escape an unpleasant life at home with their parents. Maria, a patient at the county tuberculosis sanatorium, was seventeen when she was hospitalized. "Just before I came to the sanatorium," she reported, "I was planning to get married to get away from home, but I come here instead. I'm already glad I didn't get married because I wasn't in love with the boy—I didn't even like him very much."

Common-law marriages between young people are frowned on, but it is generally known and accepted that some older couples have lived together for years without legal ceremony. Consuela and José, a middle-aged couple, lived together for ten years before they were legally married. Consuela's common-law marriage has not stigmatized her in any way in the community. She is active in the Catholic church and is well accepted by the people of the barrio.

It is expected that widowers and widows will remarry, but second marriages of divorced persons are regarded, at least temporarily, as minor scandals among both Catholic and some Protestant families. Once such a marriage is an accomplished fact, however, the couple receive gradual social acceptance.

After marriage the husband and wife usually move into a house of their own, unless there is a particular reason for them to live somewhere else. Some young men bring their wives to live with them in their parents' home if they are financially unable to set up housekeeping themselves and if their parents can afford to take on the added expense. As soon as a couple can afford to get a house, however, they usually move out.

Sometimes a young man brings his bride to his parents' home because his parents need financial help. In 9 of the 70 homes of Sal si Puedes barrio, a married son and his wife shared the house with the husband's parents. Less frequently (3 out of 70 households), young couples live with the wife's parents.

There is no appreciable difference in the relative incidence of separation and divorce among Anglos and Mexican-Americans in Mayfair. Generally there is more separation and less divorce among Spanish-speaking people than is found in Anglo groups.[6] The grounds most commonly cited for divorce are that the husband fails to provide for his wife and children or drinks to excess, or both. A few separations are caused by the deportation of one of the pair (usually the husband) from the United States as an illegal immigrant. In

---

[6] This information was furnished by a Mexican-American attorney in San Jose whose law practice acquaints him with the details of many marital disputes.

some of these separations the deportation of the husband has led to permanent termination of a marriage, and in others a temporary one.

THE AGED

Since most Sal si Puedes women continue to bear children until the time of menopause, parents usually do not finish rearing their own children until they are in their fifties or early sixties. Only parents whose children are grown and married are considered *viejitos*, elderly people.

The Spanish-speaking families of Sal si Puedes are generally devoted to the old, and it is thought that all families should take care of their elderly members. Except in rare instances, there is no feeling that having aged relatives in the home is a burden or a sacrifice. Ramón, a young father in his late twenties, maintained that there were three ways in which a man could provide old-age security for himself: "He can go get his pension if he is eligible, he can save money when he is young and buy rent property, and he can raise some good children to help him when he is old."

Both men and women work as long as they are physically fit. Even aged parents who live with their children contribute what labor they can toward the needs of the family. Doña Isabel, at eighty-one, worked in the apricot drying sheds in the summer of 1955. Her daughter commented: "*Mamacita* wouldn't have to work—we can pay her expenses all right—but she hates to stay around the house doing nothing and would rather be busy." In addition to her wage labor during the harvest season, Doña Isabel sometimes earns extra money by selling her beautiful crocheted doilies and table covers.

Barrio residents criticize young people who do not provide homes for their aged parents. Mexican-American people are generally horrified at the common American practice of sending aged relatives to sanitariums or nursing homes when they become ill or senile. Teresa advanced the theory that "when a person gets very old and has to have someone to take care of him, it is better for him to be at home with his family than in a hospital among strangers. When someone gets old, he may act a little crazy, and he needs his family with him to understand him and help him. In a hospital or a sanitarium he would only feel worse because he would think that everybody had deserted him." Elvira worked for several months as a practical nurse at a private nursing home for the aged. She reported, "Almost all the patients are old American ladies who are a little crazy. There are about twenty of them there, and only three or four have regular visitors. Others are visited by their families only once a week or even less. I think that's just terrible. They are such nice old people and they are completely neglected by their families. Their relatives just stick them in the hospital and forget about them. They could be taken care of at home just as well and would be much happier with their children and grandchildren. A few are too sick to be at home, but the least their relatives could do is to visit them regularly; someone should come every day."

De Treviño [14] expressed an opinion of Mexican family life which Mexican-Americans in Sal si Puedes share:

There is much to be gained by the presence of grandfather or grandmother. Small children learn the habit of deference to their elders, for they see their parents respectfully take this attitude. . . . Nobody supposes that young children are injured by the presence in the home of the old, senile or even slightly demented. On the contrary, they learn that we all grow old and feeble. This is reality. And they are taught compassion and patience.

DEATH AND BURIAL

The people of Sal si Puedes share the belief common in Mexico that certain birds, particularly the owl, portend imminent death.[7] Ismael related, "On the night that my mother died a big night owl came and perched on the roof of the house. It screeched and flapped its wings and wouldn't let anybody leave the house until after my mother was dead. If anybody tried to leave while she was dying, the owl would flop around and make a big racket and scare them back inside."

Paula mentioned the black hen as a bird of evil omen: "Lots of times when people are going to die, a black hen will come up to the house and crow just like a rooster. You can always tell when somebody is going to die in a house, because the house creaks and makes funny noises."

---

[7] Parsons [34] reported that in the Mexican village of Mitla, "the owl is a sign of death if it is heard at midnight; not if it is heard in the morning. Angelica says it is a sign of death only if someone is already sick. . . . Among the Aztecs if an owl perched on the house of a sick man his demise was considered certain. . . . Here they hold the belief that the barn-owl . . . is commissioned to give notice when a man is about to die. The barn-owls go to fetch the souls."

Barrio families follow a combination of Mexican and American funerary customs. When a person is thought to be dying, a priest is called (or a minister in Protestant families). The priest administers the last rites, anointing various parts of the body with holy oil. As soon as the deceased is pronounced dead, someone calls a mortuary and the body is removed immediately for embalming. After the corpse is prepared for burial and placed in a coffin (white for children, other shades—usually black—for adults), a *velorio* or wake is held.

Wakes may be held at a church, at a funeral parlor, or at home. Ordinarily, families believe that a wake should last for at least two days and two nights, but it is not always possible to have them that long. If the body is kept at the mortuary, relatives and friends are allowed to stay with the corpse only from eight to ten o'clock on two consecutive nights. This is a general rule of all local mortuaries. Because of this time limitation, most families prefer to have wakes at the church or at home. On some occasions there are funeral feasts held after the burial.

Many adults are members of burial societies which have large memberships of Spanish-speaking persons from all parts of the San Jose colony. These societies, or funerarias, are nondenominational, and both Catholics and Protestants may belong to the same group. When a member of the funeraria dies, all other members are notified of the death and are invited to attend funeral services. All members are expected to attend the wake of a deceased member and, if possible, to help with the arrangements and comfort the relatives. The various burial societies contribute different amounts—average is $300 per member—toward funeral expenses.

Catholic funerary mass or Protestant funeral services are much like those held in Anglo churches. There is the same profusion of wreaths, funeral sprays, and cut flowers which characterize American funerals. In Catholic families a rosary is said by friends and relatives of the deceased for nine nights (*la novena*) following death.

Sal si Puedes people tell many stories of having seen apparitions or ghosts of the dead. Some of the ghostly manifestations are reported to have been seen shortly after a death. Julio told the following story: "About six months ago I was driving my wife and some of her relatives home from the funeral of her cousin. Driving along Willow Street at night, I looked out and suddenly I saw a white shadowy thing that was shaped either like a coffin or like the top of an automobile. It wasn't there one minute and the next minute it was there—it floated across the street in front of the car and then disappeared. My wife's niece who was sitting in the back seat of the car saw it too. There were five other people in the car, but nobody else saw it."

Alicia told another story: "Once my brother-in-law, Trine, was driving to Los Angeles to bring me and my mother back to San Jose. Trine's brother had died a few weeks before that. As he was driving along the road, all of a sudden he heard his brother talking to him from the seat right next to him. He said his brother rode quite a ways with him and talked to him, but he was too scared to turn around and look. He knew his voice, though—it was him all right."

FAMILY STRUCTURE

Many households in Sal si Puedes are composed of nuclear or biological families, that is, a couple and their unmarried children. The nuclear family is considered the ideal living group; barrio people agree that a married couple should live in a house of their own if they can afford it. In reality, however, many households are of types other than the simple nuclear family. In 1955 a group of fifty Sal si Puedes homes were found to have the following compositions:

Households	Number
Normal nuclear families (couple and unmarried children)	23
Nuclear families plus unmarried children of one spouse by previous marriage	4
Joint families (two family heads sharing one residence) .	9
Extended families (nuclear family plus other dependents)	8
Irregular families (one of spouses absent from the home) .	4
Single-person households	2
Total households	50

In addition to the joint families listed above, a number of nuclear families who were related by kinship were found to share part of the living quarters of a related family. For example, Domingo and Ana Marquez live with their five unmarried children in a five-room house. Domingo's two married sons and their families live in a small duplex on the rear of the Marquez house lot. Rudolfo, the oldest son, and his wife and their four children live in a two-room apartment on one side of the duplex; Domingo's second son, daughter-in-law, and grandchild occupy a one-room efficiency apartment on the other side of the duplex. All three families, sixteen persons in all, share the bathroom in Domingo's house. Rudolfo's wife does most of her cooking in her own apartment on a two-burner gas hotplate, but she keeps perishable foods in the refrigerator in her mother-in-law's kitchen and sometimes uses Ana's oven for baking. All of Domingo's grandchildren frequently gather in their grandparents' living room in the late afternoon to watch television programs. While the pistol shots of cowboys and rustlers ring out in the Marquez parlor, Domingo and his sons may escape to the comparative quiet of Rudolfo's apartment to listen to the news or the ball game on the radio, and Doña Ana chats with her daughters-in-law and rocks her youngest grandchild to sleep on the other side of the duplex. Even though the three nuclear families have separate dwellings, the apartments of the married sons function simply as extensions of the paternal household. The children of the kinship group freely come and go from one house to another, feeling equally at home in all. On a warm midsummer afternoon a grandchild may fall asleep on his grandmother's bed, wake up in time to go bicycle riding with his thirteen-year-old uncle, and arrive home in time to eat supper in his aunt's apartment.

Mike, one of Domingo's grandsons, was once taken for a drive through one of San Jose's more fashionable suburbs. He saw the big brick houses, the expanses of lawn, and the high redwood fences. "I sure am glad I don't live here," he asserted; "The houses are so far apart—must be pretty lonesome!"

SPOUSES

Beals [4] has pointed out that

One of the very pervasive patterns of Latin American culture is that of male dominance and its concomitants. The father is the head of the family, woman's place is in the home as a wife and mother, and unmarried girls tend to be secluded. . . . Not only does the father have much authority in the family, but the oldest son dominates the younger. . . . Men do not entertain their friends at home but rather meet on the street or plaza, or at clubs, cantinas, restaurants, coffee shops, or pool halls. A dual standard of morality is found in which men are rather expected to have amorous adventures. . . . Women are expected to be homekeepers and to be virtuous or else bad women. . . . In the home, disciplinary control tends to be exerted solely by the father or older brother. The mother frequently does not even attempt control or correction, even to the point of not asking a small boy to close the door.

Although the patriarchal-authoritarian family pattern described above is regarded by many Sal si Puedes people as an ideal, actual family relationships in the barrio are often quite different. Wives, for example, although theoretically subservient to their husbands, sometimes openly defy male authority. Pete told the following story about his wife, Sara: "When I first came to San Jose in 1944, my brother-in-law and I got jobs at a cannery. One day on our way to work we passed by a movie and decided to go in. In those days [during World War II], they had a hard time getting men, so we didn't think that we would get fired. But when we didn't show up at work, the foreman called my wife to ask where we were. And do you know what she did? She took the bus downtown and looked until she found us and told us to go to work—so we left and went to work. I didn't even get to see all the show."

Husbands most frequently control family finances, but in some households wives exert considerable influence over purchases. Ismael and his wife, Paula, owned two cars, an old model sedan and a pickup truck. In 1955 Ismael decided that he wanted to buy a new car. He planned to trade in both his old vehicles on a new automobile and told Paula of his plan. Paula replied that he could buy a new car if he wanted to, but he was not to trade in the pickup, but should keep it for a work car. Ismael argued that he then would not have enough money to make a down payment on the new car and that he wanted to make the purchase immediately. Paula flatly vetoed her husband's plan and instructed him to save the additional money he needed and postpone buying a new car until he had accumulated enough capital. Ismael finally agreed to Paula's plan, and they remained a two-car family. "My wife has always been bossy," Ismael said with a grin; "It's worse than being in the army!"

One of Paula's neighbors, Carmen, on the other hand, has very little to say about how family money is spent. Carmen's married daughter reported the following incident: During the summer of 1955, Carmen and her four younger children contracted with a

San Jose grower to pick prunes. Carmen's husband, José, had a non-agricultural job and so was not a part of the prune-picking crew. At the end of the prune season, Carmen received a check from the grower which was $150 less than the amount that Carmen expected to be paid. Carmen had kept records of all the boxes of prunes that her family had picked each day, and she added up these figures again and again, but her records still showed that she was $150 short. Carmen asked José about the descrepancy, and he told her that she must have made a mistake. She finally went to see the prune grower to ask him to make up the difference in pay, and discovered that José and his brother had gotten a series of advance payments on the labor contract (the grower had receipts to show that the funds had been disbursed) for exactly the amount that the final check was short. Both José and his brother are fond of drinking, and Carmen discovered that they had spent the entire $150 drinking and having a good time while Carmen and her children were picking prunes.

Carmen was placed in an embarrassing situation because her husband had lied to her and told her he knew nothing about the money. She had taken him at his word and had spread the story all over the barrio of how she had been cheated by the prune grower. When Carmen finally discovered the truth, she was ashamed to admit to anyone except her daughter what had actually happened. She told her friends and neighbors simply that the matter had been settled. For weeks Carmen was furious with José, not so much for spending the money as for placing her in a ridiculous light. Finally, though, she recovered her good spirits and with a sigh of resignation commented to her daughter, "That's just the way men are."

As more barrio wives seek temporary or full-time employment outside the home, more women take an active part in planning family financial expenditures and regulating family activities. Fidel's wife, Luisa, commented, "The men are not the only important ones in the way that families live; the women have a lot to do with it. In the homes of our people, the wives and mothers are the ones who really keep the old customs and old ways alive. I think the reason that our people here in San Jose get along so well with the Anglos is because so many of us work in the canneries with Anglo women. The main reason that our people want to learn the American ways is because the women are always meeting American women at their jobs."

The change toward a more equal relationship between spouses is not always apparent to Anglo observers, however. It is true that many Sal si Puedes wives are devoted to their husbands and are frequently dependent on them in many respects. But the affection and dependency that wives feel toward their husbands find at least some counterpart in the attitudes of men toward their wives.

Although many men in the barrio follow the Mexican pattern of meeting their friends outside the home in cantinas and restaurants, there are some who invite their male friends to their homes for a bottle of beer or a game of cards. When a husband and his friends are talking in the house, however, wives and children usually discreetly retire to another part of the house in deference to the man's desire for privacy. It is expected that husbands may have flirtations with women other than their wives, and few wives express much concern about their husbands' extramarital activities as long as they are "not serious" and are handled with discretion. Men, on the other hand, are often inordinately jealous of their wives, even sometimes threatening them with violence if their suspicions are aroused.

Spouses in Sal si Puedes seldom display signs of affection for each other in public. Public demonstrations of marital devotion are generally considered bad form. On one occasion Ismael and his wife, Paula, were taking a Sunday afternoon drive in the country near San Jose. Suddenly Ismael said, "Here, mother, hold my hand—I have something that I forgot to tell you." He went on to report that the previous day his truck had turned over and that he had been trapped inside the cab for four hours. Ismael said, "I forgot all about telling you until just now." Paula's only remark to her husband was, "So you forgot to tell me, huh?" The next day, however, Paula confided to a friend, "I had to take aspirins and go to bed after we got home; I was really nervous after what Ismael told me— but don't let him know what I told you. He's spoiled enough already."

PARENTS AND CHILDREN

Although many of the aspects of parent-child relationships have been presented in the discussion of childhood and adolescent activities, it should be emphasized that in almost every Sal si Puedes family both fathers and mothers express deep affection and concern for their children. However, outward displays of sentiment on the part of parents are usually confined to very young children. Esteban, who in everyday life is somewhat formal and abrupt with his eight-year-old son, described his feelings for the boy in this way: "Last year my wife and I decided to take a trip to Tijuana. We were gone just a few days, but we had a miserable time because we both cried and cried all the time because we didn't have Davey with us. You should have seen me—man, I was really chicken!"

Both mothers and fathers have a good deal of authority over pre-adolescent children. While the father is away at work, the mother is the authority in the family. Mothers may punish very small children, but avoid administering physical punishment to older ones if possible. Even though mothers seldom administer physical punishment, children are strictly under her orders. If a mother reports to her husband that a child should be disciplined, the father nearly always unquestioningly administers the punishment posthaste. Later he may or he may not ask to be told the reason for it. Some women complain that they are unable to control their children properly because the father may work until late in the evening, returning home only after the children are in bed for the night. "The kids have the idea they can get by with anything," Marta reported. "Pete [her husband] usually stops on his way home from work and drinks beer with his friends, and all the time I'm waiting for him to come home so he can spank the kids. But when their father gets home too late, they are already asleep and I can't wake them up for a spanking. Then when morning comes and I tell Pete what the kids have done, he usually says, 'Well, it's too late to do anything about it now.'"

Some fathers are harsh disciplinarians, others tend to be more permissive with their children. This contrast was illustrated by Alfonso's comments about his compadre's behavior toward his sons: "Esteban is always afraid that his oldest boy is getting to be a problem child because the boy's teacher at school has a hard time controlling him. But I think the main problem is the way that Esteban handles the boy. Esteban is afraid that the boy will grow up to be a delinquent, and his idea of how to avoid it is to be as tough on the kid as he can. He's so afraid the kid will be spoiled that he goes overboard the other way."

Sal si Puedes fathers are generally loved and respected by their children. Ramón emphasized the importance of a father in a family: "Fathers can either make or break their kids. They can encourage them to stay in school, or if they're not the right kind of guys they can let their kids run wild. If there's no father around the house, there is no respect for the family, especially if there are girls. Everybody is coming around doing wrong things and the whole family goes mad. The same thing happens if the husband is a drunkard and doesn't ever stay at home with his family."

The oldest son of a family, especially after he reaches adolescence, may have considerable authority. Joe told the following story about his own family: "We always had trouble at home about dating. My older sister wanted to go out on dates, but my mother wouldn't let her go. She finally told my mother that she was going anyway, and she did go out. Then Mother called her cheap, said she was no good, and gave her a beating. After this trouble had gone on for a while, my oldest brother, who was a year younger than my sister, decided to step in. He stood up for my sister, and told our mother that he thought his sister should be allowed to go out on dates since it was the custom here and it didn't mean anything except having a good time. Finally my father agreed that my brother was right, and then my mother accepted the idea. Mother didn't say anything else to my sister after that; even a mother won't dispute her oldest son."

The influence that an oldest son may have even over his father is illustrated in a story that Pío told: "I've been noticing a big change in Pete lately. It began about three or four weeks ago when Pete had an argument with his oldest son, Danny [fifteen years of age]. Danny asked his father one evening for some money to take to school. He needed it for some sort of class collection. Pete told him he couldn't have the money, that they didn't have money to throw away on things like that. Danny got real mad and told his father, 'You won't let me have money for school, but you've got plenty of money to go out and get drunk on and raise hell with your buddies!' I guess Danny really gave his old man an argument, told him he was just a drunk and didn't care anything about the family. Pete took that pretty hard, and he didn't try to punish Danny for getting out of line."

"After that," Pío reported, "Pete stopped bringing home a bottle of wine every night and stopped going out to the bars so much. I guess he just needed something like his oldest son calling him a drunk to wake him up."

BROTHERS AND SISTERS

"It's a sad thing," said Paula, "when a child has no brothers or sisters. You can't keep a child like that at home—he is always leaving the house to try to find some other kids to play with. Large families are much nicer because even though they fight all the time when they're growing up, when they get older they love each other."

Parents encourage older siblings to develop a sense of responsibility toward younger children in the family. An older child has authority over a younger one, but he is also held responsible by his parents for seeing that the younger child is protected from harm and kept out of mischief. An older child may be punished if a younger brother or sister who is in his care misbehaves.

Because older children have authority over younger ones, an older sibling, particularly an older brother, may be feared by his juniors. Marta reported, "My daughter Betty [aged eleven] has the job of washing the dishes for the family. Sometimes she doesn't want to do it, but when her oldest brother, Danny, is around she goes ahead and washes them. She knows she's got a little stepfather. Danny is mean to her if she doesn't do right. He's pretty mean to all the kids, and they really work when he is around." The term little "stepfather" (*padrastrito*) is frequently applied to an older brother in Sal si Puedes.

When thirteen-year-old Mike was arrested for petty theft and was in juvenile hall in San Jose, "He just kept crying and crying and nobody could make him stop," his mother said. "That was because Mike knew that his brother [aged fifteen] was going to hit him for getting in trouble with the juvenile. He was really scared."

In spite of the authoritarian relationship between older and younger siblings, brothers and sisters are usually proud of each other and indirectly demonstrate their feelings of affection. Rosa, for example, told the story of how she had postponed her marriage for several years after her mother died "because I felt like I had to take care of my younger brothers and sisters. I wanted them to stay in school, and I just couldn't leave them alone." Four-year-old Ricky also expressed pride and affection for a younger sibling, his three-year-old brother: "I got a pretty nice little brother, talks good, knows plenty bad words!"

EXTENDED FAMILIES

Barrio people frequently have many relatives outside the nuclear family living in the San Jose area. Alicia and Esteban, for example, who have only one child of their own, are members of a kinship group of 205 persons living in Santa Clara County. Of these, 130 are Alicia's relatives and 75 are Esteban's. The couple visits frequently with about two-thirds of the members of this extended kinship group and sees the others at least two or three times a year. Alicia is in contact at least once a week, either by personal visit or by telephone conversation, with more than 60 relatives besides her husband and child.

Relations between grandparents and grandchildren are particularly close. Grandchildren respect their grandparents and are generally less formal with them than they are with their own parents. Often grandparents joke and play with their grandchildren, and demonstrations of affection are more frequent on the part of grandparents than parents. Grandmothers fondle their grandchildren and praise them in public; mothers ordinarily do not behave this way toward their own children.

Fourteen-year-old Tony and his family live in a house a few doors from Tony's grandparents. Tony's grandfather frequently asks Tony's father to send the boy over to help with some task. The father then sends Tony over to work. "I used to go over there almost every day," Tony reported. "I would work around the garden or on the house, clean the yard, or go with my grandfather somewhere in the car. Working for my grandfather is different from working for somebody else. If it gets real hot, he tells me to get in the shade or to rest for a while. My grandfather doesn't pay me, but when he gets his wages he tells my grandmother to buy me a shirt or a pair of pants. If I want to go somewhere, I can usually get the money from my grandfather, and sometimes he brings me a present. Sometimes when I'm working on my bike, my grandfather comes over to keep me company. Once I lived with my grandparents for a year, and my grandmother is just like another mother."

Relations with aunts and uncles tend to be somewhat formal and very respectful. "Cousins can always joke and have fun together.

I think it's bad that some of the younger people have begun to take their own cousins as compadres. This isn't so good because they are used to being very informal with each other and joking, arguing, or even fighting with each other. Sometimes they forget that their cousin is also their compadre or comadre and they must be very respectful toward each other."

Children are often sent to live with aunts, uncles, or grandparents for several months, or even a year, at a time. Teresa reported that her twelve-year-old daughter had been away from home for several weeks. "My daughter-in-law got lonesome with only a small baby around the house, and she wanted to keep the girl for a month or two for company."

Children live and mature in a wide circle of kinsmen. When a child feels mistreated at home, there are grandparents to comfort and console him; aunts may help him to resolve conflicts with his parents; uncles bring presents or give him a little extra spending money; cousins can always be found to share in a game or an outing; childhood secrets can be shared with older sisters; and a little boy who has a big brother need not fear the neighborhood bully. It is the rare person, whether young or old, who feels lonely in Sal si Puedes.

COMPADRAZGO

Compadrazgo, or the compadre system, is an artificial kinship complex based on various Catholic rituals and the subsequently formed relationship between a child's parents and his godparents. At the time of Catholic baptism, for example, a godfather (*padrino*) and a godmother (*madrina*) are chosen to sponsor the child for this sacrament. The godparents thus enter into a special social and religious relationship not only with their new godchild (*ahijado*) but also with the child's parents, who become their compadres. Thus, when Mike and Elvira Chavez asked Juan and Lola Martinez to serve as godparents at the baptism of the new Chavez baby, the two couples became compadres or "coparents" and thus assumed certain social and economic obligations toward each other.

Compadrazgo is a significant social institution throughout the Catholic folk cultures of southern Europe and Latin America. God-parenthood extends the size of the adult group from which a child can expect help and support; and compadrazgo links adults with one another "in bonds of mutual respect and trust . . . or, at the least, it solemnizes and sanctifies a relation of intimacy and trust that has already come into existence through . . . friendship" [39].

The compadre system is one of the strongest Mexican culture patterns found in Sal si Puedes; it plays a major role in fostering and maintaining the social stability of the community by creating new ties in the network of social relationships which bind group members together.

In Sal si Puedes four types of godparents are recognized for the following sacraments: baptism, first communion, confirmation, and marriage. Baptismal godparents are considered the most important. Their religious function is to make sure that the godchild receives proper Catholic religious instruction and all the sacraments. Their social obligations to the child are to see that he does not lack the necessities of life and to supply goods and money, if the parents are unable to provide them, for the child's rearing. In Sal si Puedes, however, these obligations are more ideal than real.

Baptismal godparents, as well as other kinds of godparents, are expected to give their godchild gifts at Christmas, on his birthday, at the time of his marriage, and at the time of his confirmation. They are expected to give advice and administer discipline to the child whenever they deem it necessary, with or without the invitation of the parents. It is generally agreed in Sal si Puedes that a child is more likely to heed advice from a godparent than from his own parents. Although godparents are supposed ideally to administer religious instruction, very few in Sal si Puedes exercise this function.

Relations Between Compadres

The relationship between compadres is a warm and friendly one, but it is believed that compadres should not tease or joke with each other. Above all they should not argue or fight. Marta commented, "My third son is going to take his first communion next month. I don't have a padrino for him yet. I'd like to get Ismael, but he's always teasing me and telling me jokes, so I guess I'll have to get somebody else for the padrino."

Compadres are considered as close as blood relatives and any sort of sexual relationship between them is strictly forbidden. As Rosa said, "Even if the woman's husband died and her compadre's wife died, they could never marry or have anything to do with each other—it would be just as bad as marrying your brother." This prohibition, however, does not extend to the compadre's relatives, even those of his nuclear family.

Compadres visit each other frequently, usually several times a week, and assist each other with labor whenever an extra pair of hands is needed. Irene stated, "I'm really lucky to have one of my comadres living right across the street from me. It gives me someone to visit and to go with me when I want to go out. I wouldn't feel right about asking just anybody to go somewhere with me, but I know I can always ask my comadre."

Two women who are comadres often give each other small presents—a dish of some delicacy which one has prepared, a potted plant, a bit of embroidery or crocheted lace. If one needs to borrow a cup of flour or a few beans, the person to ask is, naturally, a comadre. A woman will not hesitate to leave her husband and children to prepare their own dinner in order to go to the aid of a comadre who needs help. When Paula's comadre, who lives in Hayward (about twenty-five miles from San Jose), was expecting her last baby, Paula left her own family for two weeks to care for her comadre during her confinement.

Men render whatever financial help they can to their compadres who are having economic problems. Pete said, "I sure would like to get my compadre Chavez in the plant where I work; he hasn't got a job right now."

Esteban's story illustrates the fact that a man may feel obligated to help a compadre even if the compadre has relatives who are in a position to come to his aid: "I have always felt like being a compadre was a serious thing and placed me under obligation to do the best I could. Take my compadre Raphael, for example. I was the godfather at his son's wedding. Now Raphael is old and has lost his wife. He lives on a little pension. He has two stepsons living, but those guys don't take their responsibilities seriously, and they didn't ask Raphael to come and live with them after their mother died. So my wife and I talked it over and decided to ask Raphael to come and live with us. He's an old man and he gets pretty lonesome without any family around. I wouldn't have felt right if I hadn't asked him to live here—after all, he is my compadre."

Social Functions of the Compadre System

Compadrazgo in Sal si Puedes serves three main social functions: it formalizes friendship and extends the size of the kinship group, it enhances neighborhood solidarity, and if compadres are also members of the extended family it strengthens kinship ties.

During 1954 and 1955, Elvira became very friendly with another woman of the barrio, Manuela. Manuela lived across the street from Elvira's mother; she and Elvira both were members of the Sociedad Guadalupana (Altar Society), and both had children of about the same ages. During the summer of 1955, two of Elvira's children were to take their first communion, and Elvira was able to ask Manuela to sponsor her daughter and Manuela's husband to act as communion godfather for her son. Thus the couple became Elvira's compadres, but not through the same child. "I'm real happy," Elvira remarked; "Manuela and I have been such good friends the last couple of years. Now I know that we will always be friends no matter what happens." The compadre system served to formalize friendship and to create a permanent bond between people who wanted to retain that friendship.

The role of compadrazgo in neighborhood solidarity is illustrated by the experience of Pete and Marta. In the winter of 1954, this couple and their children moved from a nearby barrio to Sal si Puedes. After they had lived in their present home for about six months, Marta had a new baby. She asked her new neighbors to the east to serve as baptismal godparents for the child and thus entered into a compadre relationship with them. A few months later the family's eleven-year-old daughter was to be confirmed in the Catholic Church. Pete and Marta decided to ask another neighbor, the woman whose house was next door to theirs on the west, to sponsor the girl in her confirmation. Thus, within a year Pete and Marta had set up close relations with two families living adjacent to them. "Now that I have comadres living nearby," Marta explained, "I really feel at home in this house."

There is a tendency in Sal si Puedes for people to select at least a few of their compadres from among their own relatives. Since Mexican-American families in the barrio are large and since each older child may have several godparents, a single individual may have as many as eight or ten compadres living in his immediate neighborhood; of these, most are usually nonrelatives but are generally related to him in some way. Frequently a child's uncle or aunt is asked to become the child's godparent; thus brothers and sisters may also be compadres. Cousins are frequently chosen also.

Rosa emphasized the function of the compadre system in family solidarity: "I think having relatives as compadres is a pretty good thing sometimes because it makes distant relatives like aunts, uncles, and cousins seem much closer, and it keeps the family from drifting apart."

7

SICKNESS AND HEALTH

THE ADULT population of Sal si Puedes barrio is composed in the main of first- and second-generation Mexican-Americans. Most of them or their parents entered the United States during the first thirty years of this century, bringing with them medical beliefs and practices from Mexican towns and villages. Rural Mexico had at that time been little influenced by the scientific medical practice which has now been extended to many parts of the country.

When Juana's parents entered the United States in 1910, immunization for diphtheria was unknown, the relation of insulin to diabetes was undiscovered, and there was no known cure for rickets. During the years of Mexican-American residence in the United States, language barriers, low social and economic status, settlement in semi-isolated colonies, and other factors have proved impediments to free communication and social intercourse with English-speaking people. In the early days of Mexican immigration and settlement, few messengers brought to the barrios of San Jose news of the startling medical discoveries being made. The people dreaded illness, prayed for good health, and attacked disease with the only weapons they had—the herbal remedies and traditional curing practices of village Mexico.

Folk concepts of disease from Mexico are still important to Mexican-Americans; many of these beliefs persist in the thinking of second- and third-generation Americans and in many ways continue to influence their health behavior.

The medical beliefs and practices in Sal si Puedes are described in the following pages. Sections are devoted to the theories and practices of folk medicine and the nature of medical relations between barrio people and health workers.

FOLK MEDICINE

The term "folk curing" as it is used here refers to those therapeutic practices which are derived from Mexican patterns and based on the various "folk theories" of disease described in the following pages. Folk cures may be administered by anyone who has the requisite knowledge: a patient may treat himself, may ask a friend or relative who "knows herbs and other cures" to perform treatments or prepare medicines for him, or may go to a curandera—a specialist in the diagnosis and treatment of folk syndromes. Curanderas expect to be paid a small fee for their services. There is no idea that curing women have unusual or supernatural powers; they are simply those who have more than the usual lay knowledge of the lore of Mexican folk medicine. There is not a clear distinction between curanderas and women who "know a little curing." Paula, for example, is regarded as a curandera by several barrio people. She herself, however, said: "I don't know why you think I'm a curandera; I just know a little about herbs." Since it is impossible to distinguish curing women from those who "know a little curing," no effort has been made in the following pages to differentiate cures administered by folk practitioners from "home remedies."

Folk therapy consists of oral administration of various herbs and purgatives; topical application of liniments, oils, and herbal mixtures; massage (*sobadas*); "cupping" (*ventosas*); regulation of the diet; and magical cures. Any one or a combination of these may be used for a particular syndrome.

Since the treatment of a disease depends on the etiological theory associated with it, both causative and curative beliefs are discussed in each of the following groups of common "folk diseases."

THEORY OF DISEASE

Ideas about disease and its causes are varied in Sal si Puedes. Some concepts are clearly derived from Mexican folk beliefs and others are "scientific" syndromes recognized in both Mexico and the United States. Although barrio people themselves have no clear-cut classification of pathologies, diseases well known to them are grouped here, for purposes of organization, into the following categories: diseases of "hot and cold" imbalance, diseases of dislocation of internal organs, diseases of magical origin, diseases of emotional origin, other folk-defined diseases, and "standard scientific" diseases.

It is not always easy to place a disorder in a single category. For example, there are mechanical injuries such as burns which are clearly traumatic but which also are thought to cause an imbalance of body temperature. Other syndromes are thought to be primarily magical in origin (for example, *mal aire*), but disturbances in "hot and cold" may make the victim particularly susceptible to the disorder. The etiology of even the "standard scientific" diseases may be misunderstood and the disorder attributed to magical causes.

Diseases of "Hot and Cold" Imbalance

The "hot and cold" theory of disease is derived from the Hippocratic theory of pathology, which postulated that the human body in a state of health contained balanced quantities of the four "humours" (phlegm, blood, black bile, and yellow bile). Some of the four "humours" were thought to be innately "cold." A disproportion of hot and cold body essences was reflected in illness. This body of belief was brought to the New World by sixteenth-century Spanish explorers and colonists and was widely diffused among the native inhabitants of Spanish-America [18]. Foster and Rowe [20] have pointed out that

Ethnologists have found in many parts of Latin America that important ideas concerning health and sickness are based on the Graeco-Roman concept of "hot" and "cold" qualities innate in nature; for example, certain illnesses are believed to be inherently "hot," and are treated with "cold" remedies, while other illnesses are "cold" and are treated with "hot" remedies. Food also is often so classified, and the maintenance of health requires care to avoid mixing of incompatible dishes. The qualities of "hot" and "cold" in this system have nothing to do with physical temperature and nothing necessarily to do with physiological effect. . . . The attribution of a substance to one or the other of these categories may be purely arbitrary.

Although there is a good deal of reliance placed on diet modification for illness, there are relatively few people who know which foods are "hot" and which are "cold." Most know about a few foods (chilies, pork, tomatoes, citrus fruits, watermelons), but only about one-third of barrio adults were able to classify other foods. Table 8 lists the "hot" and "cold" designations assigned to some common foods in Sal si Puedes.

Dietary regulation is thought vital to good health, and many disorders are traced to imbalanced intake of "hot" and "cold" foods or to the ingestion at the same meal of foods which are extreme opposites in heat and cold. Fidel's wife, for example, attributed his upset stomach to the latter: "People really have to be careful what they eat because it's easy to get an upset stomach if you eat bad combinations of food such as hot chilies with cold foods, especially cold beer. You have to be very careful what you eat with any dish containing *chiles bravos* [extremely hot red peppers]."

There is a tendency to think less in terms of the "qualities" of "hot" and "cold" and more in terms of actual temperature of foods. For example, Fidel's wife advised against eating "hot" chilies with "cold" beer—yet beer is almost everywhere in Mexico regarded as a "hot" food. With the decrease in popular knowledge of "hot and cold" designations, there is a corresponding decrease in the therapeutic use of foods. "Hot and cold" disorders are coming to be treated more frequently with herbal remedies or with topical applications which either warm or cool the affected area (the latter again reflecting the general confusion between "innate qualities" and actual physical temperatures).

The mother of a three-year-old boy attributed his head cold to eating too much watermelon, thought to be a very "cold" food. Infants and small children are believed to be unusually vulnerable to "cold stomach," an imbalance producing symptoms of colic. Babies, therefore, should not be given large quantities of such "cold" foods as melon and citrus fruits (a fact which might account for the resistance some mothers demonstrate to giving infants daily orange juice).

It is thought that some individuals are more susceptible to "hot and cold" imbalance than others. The story was told of a bracero

TABLE 8

HOT AND COLD FOODS

Food Types	Very hot	Hot	Temperate	Cold	Very cold
Vegetables	Chile pepper, green Chile pepper, red Garlic	Onion		Beans, green Beets Cabbage Carrots Cauliflower Coriander Parsley Peas Pumpkin Radish Squash Turnip	Cucumber Pickles Purslain Spinach Tomato
Meats and milk	Crackles	Capon Fish Milk, goat's Pork Turkey	Goat	Beef Boar Lamb Milk, cow's Milk, donkey's Mutton Rabbit	Hen or pullet Milk, human
Starches and sweets	Beans, white	Barley Bread, wheat Beans (habas) Chick peas Potato, Irish Potato, sweet Rice Sweet rolls Tortillas, wheat Wheat Honey Sugar, brown Salt	Beans, pinto Sugar, white	Beans, red Lentils Oatmeal Tortillas, corn Vermicelli	

from the state of Oaxaca in southern Mexico who came to San Jose to pick apricots. It was said that he wanted to save all his wages to take back to Mexico with him, so he ate nothing but apricots from the orchard for several weeks. His subsequent illness and death was attributed to his diet of "cold" fruit. It was suggested that people from such warm climates as that of Oaxaca were particularly sensitive to "cold."

Avoidance of certain items of diet during pregnancy was discussed in chapter 6. To summarize, an expectant mother should avoid eating very "hot" foods lest her child suffer from chincual (diaper rash) after it is born. Postpartum diet is strictly regulated in terms of "hot and cold" foods; thus fruit juices, tomatoes, pork, and certain fresh vegetables should be avoided because "they are too cold for the stomach" of a woman at such a critical time. Eating them produces "bumps on the legs," that is, varicose veins.

Many observers have commented on the vast number of herbal remedies that are commonly used both in Mexico and among Mexican-Americans in the United States. (For discussions of Mexican-American herbal lore, see Campa [12] and Curtin [13].) In Sal si Puedes almost every kitchen garden has a few plants whose leaves, flowers, or roots are used in the preparation of herb medicines. Several Mexican-American pharmacies keep stocks of popular Mexican herbs. Some of the most frequently mentioned medical herbs are: alfalfa, *albahaca* (sweet basil), *alcanfór* (camphor leaves), *alhucema* (lavender), *ajo* (garlic), *adormidera* (poppy seeds), *canela* (cinnamon bark), *cascara* (cascara bark), *chabacán* (apricot), *cilantro* (coriander), *clavo* (cloves), *comino* (cumin), *casia* (cassia), *eneldo* (dill), *epazote* (saltwort), *estafiate* or *estafisagria* (larkspur), *hinojo* (fennel), *hojas de limón* (lemon leaves), *manzanilla* (camomile), *mastranzo* (round-leaved mint), *flor de naranja* (orange blossoms), *orégano* (wild marjoram), *poleo* (pennyroyal), *romero* (rosemary), *rosa de castilla* (rose of Castile), *ruda* (rue), *hojas de sen* (senna leaves), *tilo* (linden), *toronjil* (balm gentle), and *yerba buena* (mint).

Herbs are used for a variety of conditions, including those thought to result from "hot" and "cold" imbalance. Rue is a favorite herb and is thought particularly effective against excessive "cold" in the body. When Paula got an earache secondary to an upper respiratory infection, she attributed it to cold air blowing in her ears. She attempted to prevent the earache from becoming more severe by stuffing leaves of fresh rue in her ears—rue (*ruda,* in Spanish) is thought to be a "hot" herb.

Alicia uses herbs to clear a stuffy nose accompanying a head cold: "For *catarro constipado,* make an infusion of *poleo, mastranzo,* and *alhucema* [pennyroyal, round-leaved mint, and lavender]. Pour some of the liquid into the cupped palm and sniff it up into the nostrils. It will clear the head and open the nose."

Factors other than imbalanced diet may produce an excess of heat or cold in the body and thus lead to illness. General credence is given the idea that cold air, particularly wind or drafts, can lead to *enfriamiento,* "catching cold" in some part of the body. ("Catching cold" is not used here in the sense of acquiring a common head cold—Spanish has a distinct word, *resfriado,* for the latter.) Victims of enfriamiento usually complain of pain in a joint, particularly the knee or shoulder. To restore the affected part to a temperate state, heat or remedies thought to contain the "quality of heat" are applied topically to the affected area. Actual increase in temperature is sometimes used also. A common cure is packing the rheumatic part in hot sand and leaving it there until it begins to sweat.

Infant colic (attributed to a "cold stomach") is treated by massaging the back and legs with warm olive oil; the oil is rubbed vigorously on the skin until a red glow appears.

Angina (tonsillitis or sore throat) is sometimes treated by rubbing the feet vigorously with Vicks VapoRub. The same treatment is given to a child who is cutting teeth. A teething child is thought especially vulnerable to "cold stomach" and at that time is expected to have mild diarrhea. One woman reported that when her grandchild began teething, "he got sad eyes and a little diarrhea —so I knew the teeth were causing a little stomach cold." Her treatment consisted of first breaking an egg on the baby's stomach; the egg was allowed to run over the abdomen until the yolk came to rest. The spot at which the yolk stopped was regarded as the seat of the trouble. She then made a paste of flour and spread it on a cloth which was bound around the child's abdomen over the "cold" place. (Wheat flour is thought to be a "hot" substance.) The plaster was left on overnight, and the next morning the grandmother reported joyfully, "Now the baby is cured."

A child who has frequent nosebleeds is thought to be "overheated" and may be given two or three cold baths a day for a period of time as a prophylaxis.

Burns of the skin are usually first treated with lard, a "cold" substance.

When Marta's younger son acquired a skin eruption, she decided it was the result of his eating too much "cold" fruit. The lesions produced a clear watery exudate (water as "cold") and were thus classified as "cold sores." Marta reported, "I put merthiolate on and that burned it all right, but it seemed to get worse anyway." Since merthiolate burns an open sore, it is thought a "hot" substance efficacious in the treatment of various "cold" disorders. When the child's rash did not respond to this treatment, Marta urged her husband to bring home some "sugar plums" (a sweet red plum) from the orchard. This "hot" fruit, she explained, is excellent for children who have skin rashes.

Ventosas, or "cupping," is thought to be a good treatment for backache or "cold" in any part of the body. Paula's procedure is to mount a small candle on the flat surface of a coin (Paula believes a copper penny is best but other people sometimes use silver). The treatment is improved if the candle is one that has been blessed at Candlemas, "but it doesn't matter because you are going to pray anyway." The coin and candle are placed over the painful spot and the candle lit. A small jar or glass is placed over the burning candle. The flame soon exhausts the air inside the glass, the candle is extinguished, and the skin is pulled up by the partial vacuum inside the glass. Paula usually recites a prayer while the candle is burning: "*Saco este dolor en el Nombre de Dios* [I draw out this pain in the name of God]." The glass is then moved around over the back, massaging the skin and drawing blood to the surface. "When the pain is drawn up into the jar," Paula reported, "you can feel it going out of your back and the relief is wonderful." After removing the apparatus, the back is rubbed with *aceite volcánico* (volcanic oil—a "hot" substance).

A school nurse reported the following case. A little boy who had had chronic earache for several months failed to improve although notices had been sent home to the parents urging them to have the child treated. Finally the mother was called to school to talk with the school physician. When the parent was told that the child's ear must be treated, she insisted that indeed he had been treated and was now cured. The "cold" in his ear, she reported, had been cured by his grandmother: she had blown hot air into it. A funnel had been placed with the tip in the ear canal and a paper torch lighted and held up before the large end of the funnel. Warm air and smoke were then blown into the ear from the burning paper via the funnel. The nurse reported that it required some persuasion to convince the mother that the child's ear was still infected.

Barrenness in women may be due to a "cold womb." A well-known *curandera* uses a combined topical and herbal treatment: "Fill a a wash tub with hot water in which is placed some romero (rosemary) and have the woman sit over the tub. The vapors will warm the womb, and the woman can then conceive a child."

Some of the other medications used as an aid to conception also involve the use of "hot" substances. Some of those thought to be most beneficial are: (1) A plaster of belladonna leaves made with a flannel cloth and placed on the back over the sacral area each morning for several consecutive days. (Belladonna plaster is sold in most pharmacies as a simple topical analgesic.) (2) A series of doses of a patent medicine, Brandreth's Pills. This medication contains a cathartic, mandrake root (*Podophyllum peltatum*), ordinarily used for chronic constipation. The pills are taken with a cup of chocolate in which a little powdered sulphur is mixed. Three pills are taken on each of three consecutive days. During this time the woman avoids all "cold" foods, drinks as little water as possible, and does not take a bath. This regimen is designed to "build up heat" in the body and thus "warm the cold womb."

Diseases of Dislocation of Internal Organs

Foster [18] has reported that "In parts of both Spain and America it is believed that illness results when real or imaginary parts of the body move from their normal positions." In Sal si Puedes the most common of these disorders is *mollera caída* ("fallen fontanelle"), which is thought to result when the "part of the head" directly under the anterior fontanelle of an infant "drops." The displaced part is thought to lie above, and form a depression in, the hard palate. The symptoms of the disease are severe diarrhea and vomiting.

Mollera caída is diagnosed by observing a depression of the anterior fontanelle. A further diagnostic procedure is examination, with the fingers, of the hard palate; if the child is affected, a *bolita* (little ball) is felt in the roof of the mouth.

Paula explained the relation between the condition and gastrointestinal symptoms: "The bolita causes the baby to be unable to nurse well because he can't close his mouth right with the bolita there. He just sucks and smacks his lips all the time but can't get enough to eat." This was the only "explanation" for the symptoms of mollera caída given in Sal si Puedes. Other people knew of the disorder but were unable to explain it. The concept of mollera seems to be based on the observed loss of subcutaneous fluid over the fontanelle—a result of the dehydration caused by infant diarrhea. There is a confusion of cause and effect in folk belief; the depressed fontanelle and the exaggeration of palatal rugae resulting from fluid loss are assumed to be primary causative factors.

Topical treatment is widely used for mollera caída. Several cures are popular in the barrio, all of them aimed at "getting the mollera back in place." An infant with the disorder may be held up by the ankles, head down, with the crown of the head dipped into a pan of tepid water. The child is suspended in this position for one to two minutes in the hope that the mollera will fall back in place. Sometimes the person conducting the treatment (usually a curandera) pounds or slaps the soles of the feet while the child is in an inverted position. Some curers recite prayers during the treatment.

Another remedy for mollera consists of applying continuous pressure to the child's hard palate with the fingertips. The curandera may also attempt to replace the fallen part by sucking on the area. This procedure was described by Manuela as follows: "Trim the hair off the baby's head right over the soft spot. Then take a mouthful of warm water, put your mouth over the mollera and suck on the spot. This may pull the mollera back in place."

Plasters may be used to cure difficult cases of mollera: "If nothing else works," Paula advised, "break an egg and take the 'nervio' [germinal tissue] of the egg and put it on a piece of cigarette paper. Plaster this over the mollera and press on it until it sticks tight. Then you can just leave it there and forget about it—the baby will get well in a few days." Teresa also advised a poultice for fallen fontanelle: "Make a thick paste of soap—a bar of yellow hand soap is the best—mixed with table sugar. Put this paste on the baby's mollera and leave it there all day. The next morning you can wash it off and put on a new plaster. You should do this every day until the mollera comes back up."

A second condition related to displacement of organs or tissues is described as the presence of "lumps or bolitas" (little balls) in the tissues of arms or legs. Irregularities of the extremities such as those formed by varicosities or ganglion masses may be attributed to "the nerves being out of place." Massage or physical manipulation of the affected part is thought to help the condition. One woman reported that massage with an electric vibrator was the best treatment.

It is thought that barrenness in women may be due to "cold womb" (see above), or it may be diagnosed as the result of a "fallen or twisted" uterus. A cure for this disorder is massage of the abdomen with oil until "the womb is put back in place."

Diseases of Magical Origin

Mal ojo, or "evil eye," is a disorder of children and infants that is thought to have a magical origin. The concept in Sal si Puedes is similar to its European and Latin-American counterpart [18]. It is believed that if someone, especially a woman, admires someone else's child and looks at him without actually touching him, the child may fall ill of ojo. Anyone can inflict evil eye upon a child, and the offending person may not even be conscious of the damage he has done. The symptoms are rather vague, but usually include some or all of the following: fitful sleep, crying a great deal without apparent cause, diarrhea, vomiting, fever (similar to the list given for mollera caída). Evil eye can be prevented if the potential culprit, after admiring a child, touches him.

The condition is diagnosed by rubbing the child's body with a whole raw egg; the egg is subsequently broken and the yolk examined. A red spot, or "eye," on the yolk is a diagnostic sign. The diagnosis of mal ojo is not common in Sal si Puedes. Most adults know of the concept, but few women in the barrio were discovered who knew the details of its diagnosis and cure.

Mal ojo is usually cured with eggs. One curandera uses the following procedure: An unbroken egg, preferably one freshly laid, is held in the curer's right hand and used to make the sign of the cross on all parts of the child's body. During this procedure the Apostles' Creed is recited three times. The egg is next broken into a small bowl of water. Six small pieces of holy palm (taken from the church on Palm Sunday) are placed to form three small crosses on top of the egg. ("If you haven't got any palm," the curer advised, "just use an ordinary broomstraw.") The sick child is put to bed and the bowl of water, egg, and palm is placed under his bed, directly beneath his head. The next morning the child is expected to be cured.

Some people report that a "sure sign that the evil eye is drawn out of the child is if you find the next morning that the egg looks cooked. Then you know the mal ojo has been drawn into the egg and the child will be all right."

Mal aire (bad air) is classified here as a magical concept because in most parts of Mexico the disease is thought to be the result of evil spirits or other vaguely conceived forces which inhabit the air and which may, under certain circumstances, possess an unsuspecting victim and cause him to fall ill.[1] In Sal si Puedes mal aire seems to be more closely related to the "hot and cold" theory of disease than to supernaturalism.

The symptoms produced by it vary, but most commonly are some sort of facial twisting or paralysis. Manuela told the following story: "Three years ago the mother of my daughter's baptismal padrino got out of her warm bed and went out into the hall, which was very cold, and then into a hot shower. Just as she came back out of the shower into the cold hall again, she said she felt just like something hit her real hard right on the forehead. Then she got a terrible pain in her head and neck. When she got back to her room, she saw that her face was crooked, her cheek drooped on one side, and her mouth was twisted up. She called her son and his wife and told them she had an attack of mal aire. She asked them to bring her some ruda [the herb, rue] mixed with warm camphorated oil and olive oil. They went all over the barrio looking for the ruda because it was at night and the drugstores were closed. They finally

---

[1] Parsons [34] reported from Mexico: "I have heard *aigre*, the air, wind, referred to as if it were an evil spirit of the air that takes possession of a person. . . . '*Aire* is like a wind. It makes a commotion in the body. It catches you suddenly, it enters the body.' You may be overheated, you go outdoors, the 'air' hits you. . . . 'From much thinking the head is heated, then the air hits. This air does harm. . . . [A patient] was described as having a violent temper . . . and at such times the 'air' strikes. . . . [when] one gets very angry, [he is] . . . subject to the 'air.'" This describes the way in which *mal aire* is conceived in Sal si Puedes, also. It is not clear whether the etiology is an evil spirit, overheating, or anger—perhaps a combination of all three.

found a bush in somebody's yard and got the fresh leaves. They mashed these in the oil and took it to the old lady. She kept rubbing in on her face and neck every few hours, and finally she got better. Now the only sign of her sickness is a little droop of one of her eyelids, so I guess the medicine was the right thing to use."

Other people had heard of mal aire but commented that "here we call it *alferecía* [epilepsy]."

Brujería, or witchcraft, is regarded as a cause of disease by many people. A local Spanish-speaking doctor whose patients are mostly Mexican-Americans estimated that about 25 per cent of his patients express a belief in witchcraft and suggest it as the cause of their illnesses.

Dolores, a twenty-five-year-old woman born in California, reported: "When I was a kid, I heard a lot of talk about *brujas* [witches], but I never believed in them until I went to visit my aunt down near Yuma, Arizona. One night I heard a racket at the window screen; I looked around and saw a big *thing* hanging on the screen. I yelled for my aunt and she came in and told me that it was a big bird—something like a *tecolote* [owl]—and that a witch had sent it there to make one of us sick. I just laughed, and told her she was crazy. She got a little mad at me and said she was going to prove something to me. So she didn't do anything until the next night—and, you know, that bird stayed right on the window screen all that time. Finally she said that if we didn't do something, somebody was really going to get sick. She got some ashes from the stove and sprinkled them in the shape of a cross at each corner of the house. Then my uncle took a little bag of salt and tied it on top of the roof. Pretty soon the owl flew up to the roof and just sat there like it was paralyzed and my uncle killed it with a shotgun. After that, none of our family got sick. But we knew there was a witch around there, all right, because a few weeks later the man next door got real sick. They took him to all kinds of doctors, but they couldn't find a thing wrong with him. He kept getting thinner and thinner until he finally died. It was that witch who killed him with brujería. Since that time, I never laugh about things like that."

Malevolent witchcraft seems to be more theory than practice in Sal si Puedes. Many people believe that witches exist who can cause illness through magical procedures. There is none, however, who is able to describe spells or hexes, and no one admits being able to practice "black magic." There were several reports about a witch living in San Jose; however, when this woman was traced, it was found that she was not engaged in sorcery but was a curandera who used some magical cures for diseases she was called upon to treat.

Spells, prayers, religious objects (as pictures of saints), and holy water may be used to ward off evil forces. It is said that barrenness may be caused by witchcraft. A famous curandera in Decoto, a town near San Jose, is said to treat barren women with keys which have been blessed by placing them before the santos (the figures in the church depicting various saints). The keys are then suspended from the waist so that they hang over the abdomen in the area of the womb. This curer is frequently asked to treat diseases attributed to witchcraft. She "used to use herbs a lot more than she does now. Lately she has been curing brujería with *agua puro* [plain water] which has been placed for a while before the images of the saints. This isn't regular holy water—she blesses it herself."

Diseases of Emotional Origin

In most parts of Latin America intense or prolonged emotional states are recognized as the source of some illnesses. Foster [17] identifies the relationship:

Folk recognition that strong emotional experiences can cause an individual to fall ill is evidenced by the wide variety of names for sicknesses that are essentially psychosomatic. The emotional experiences which most often produce physiological results include fright, anger, desire, imagined rejection, embarrassment or shame, disillusion, and sadness.

In Sal si Puedes two strong emotional states are thought of as morbid entities: fright (*susto* or *espanto*) and anger (*bilis*, literally "bile").

The term "bilis" is not always used to indicate a disease; sometimes it means simply that a person is nervous or "upset" about something. In its medical sense, however, bilis is a disorder which is diagnosed and treated like any other illness. Adults are said to be particularly susceptible to it. The illness always comes on after a person becomes very angry, especially if he flies into an uncontrollable rage. A day or two after this fit of anger, the attack occurs. The disorder produces symptoms of acute nervous tension, chronic fatigue, and malaise.

Bilis is ordinarily treated with herbal remedies. Linden leaves and balm gentle may be used prophylactically to "quiet the nerves" and prevent loss of temper. The variety of herbs which may be prescribed for a single disorder is illustrated by the following three herb medicines used as specifics against bilis.

1. A tea is made by boiling in a cup of water for several minutes three herbs: *romero, manzanilla,* and *hoja de alcanfor* (rosemary, camomile, and camphor leaf). The tea should be drunk *en ayunas* (before breakfast) on nine consecutive mornings. Most medicines and treatments are given either three or nine times; these numbers are thought to have a ritual significance.

2. Some *casia* (cassia bark), *cogollas de limón* (lemon shoots), *un limón* (a whole lemon), *canela* (cinnamon bark), and *nuez tostada* (toasted walnut) are all combined with a pint of whiskey. A half-cup of this medicine is taken en ayunas for nine consecutive mornings.

3. A third remedy for bilis utilizes the following herbs and other substances: *yerba buena* (mint), *hinojo* (fennel), *eneldo* (dill), *casia* (cassia bark), magnesium bicarbonate, *almendra de chabacán* (kernel of apricot seed), peel of a sour orange, pomegranate peel, a few drops of lemon juice, and sugar. All the ingredients are ground in a mortar (*molcajete*) with a small quantity of water and then boiled in about two cups of water for several minutes. A dose of this medicine is taken en ayunas for nine days.

Susto, or fright, is one of the most common folk diseases. A variety of symptoms are attributed to it. Alicia described it in this way: "Susto is a very bad thing to get—you can die from it. Children mostly have it. Something scares them real bad, and it seems like they just can't stop being scared from then on. When a child has susto, you can tell because he is very pale and thin and doesn't want to eat. He gets big round eyes that look sad, and he always has headaches. He shakes and trembles and is scared of the least little thing."

Rosa said, "My younger sister used to suffer from susto when she was a little girl. Whenever anything scared her, she would faint and lie unconscious for a few minutes. My mother said it was because she was frightened badly when she was pregnant with my sister, and that it would go away when my sister got older. That was right because she stopped having those fainting spells when she was about twelve years old, and she hasn't fainted since."

Paula furnished the following information about curing susto: "Susto is a hard thing to cure. It's best not to get it in the first place. Children usually get it, but if a pregnant woman is asustada [frightened], it will affect the child, and the baby will be born with susto. If a woman is expecting and gets a bad fright, she can avoid giving the baby susto by taking a remedy immediately. She should take a glass of warm water and drop into it a few live coals from the fire. Add a little sugar to this water and drink it all right away."

It is thought that susto can be cured easily if the disease is detected and treated in an early stage. One woman reported: "I cured a little girl last year, but the same treatment didn't work for my comadre's little boy because he had had susto for years before they asked me to try to cure him. After I tried the remedy, they took him to the county hospital where they tested him for TB and some other things. But they couldn't find a thing wrong with him. He had *el susto viejo* ["old fright"], and nobody can cure that."

A popular cure is as follows: "Cut two branches of leaves of a sweet-pepper tree. Take a candle and mount it in the middle of a saucer and put a little water around the candle. Light the candle and put the saucer on the floor. The child should walk across it [legs apart, one foot on each side of the saucer] in one direction, then across it again at right angles, making a cross. Then take the branches of pepper leaves and 'sweep' the child with them all over, first from top to bottom, then across from left to right, making the sign of the cross. Go on with the sweeping until you have finished reciting three *credos* [Apostles' Creed]. After this, put the child to bed with the two pepper branches laid to form a cross under the child's bed. Just as you walk away from the bed, you must call out three times: '*Vente* [child's name], *no te quieres ni te espantes* [Come, ———, you don't need anything and you aren't afraid].'" When this sentence has been recited three times, the cure is over for that night. The cure should be started on a Wednesday night just before bedtime, and must be repeated in its entirety the following two nights, Thursday and Friday, at the same hour. After the third night's treatment, it is thought that the child is cured of susto if he can be cured at all.

There are indications in the details of treatment for susto that the disease is thought somehow related to the concept of "soul loss." Foster [16] has reported that

A common primitive concept of a cause of illness is fright which jars the soul loose from the body. The result, soul loss, is the real cause of illness; fright merely accounts for the separation of the soul. Fragmentary data from several parts of Mexico suggest that soul loss from fright was at one time a popular superstition in the country . . . some traces still remain.

The treatment described above, which includes calling to the child by name ("Come here, you aren't afraid"), suggests that susto is related to soul loss in Sal si Puedes—the curandera begs the soul to return to the body. (Besides Foster, cited above, see also Gillin [23] and Redfield [39] for discussions of emotional syndromes.)

Other Folk-defined Diseases

Two conditions regarded by barrio people as disease states do not fall into any of the above categories. These are *latido* and *empacho*.

Latido (palpitation) is a folk concept, regarded as a serious, often fatal, disease.[2] The disease is thought to be caused by going without food for a long time. Elvira said, "Latido comes on when somebody doesn't eat anything for a long time—maybe two or three days. The stomach gets weak, and they get pains here in the stomach [pointing to the diaphragmatic area] and in their chest and sometimes up to their shoulders. Then, the persons can't eat even if they try. You can feel the stomach pulsate if you put your hand on it, and that's a very bad sign. Sometimes my mother will go without food for a couple of days—just take coffee and cigarettes. Then, after a day or two, she tries to eat again but she can't. The food comes back up in her throat, and she gets this latido in her stomach."

Advanced forms of latido are characterized by severe emaciation with loss of abdominal fat and an empty stomach and intestines. This makes it possible to feel the normal pulsation of the abdominal aorta on deep palpation. The pulsation is taken to be a distinct sign of the disease. A patient may be diagnosed as having latido if he is

[2] Beals [3] reported on *latido* from Mexico: "Heart trouble, *latido de corazón*, is recognized from pains in the heart and by palpitations. There is a high fever, a cough, and sometimes the patient spits blood. . . . The disease may be caused if the person arrives somewhere very agitated and drinks cold water or something cold, *fresca*."

sufficiently thin, from whatever cause, to permit feeling the abdominal aorta.

Empacho (surfeit) is characterized by the presence of a large ball in the stomach which produces swelling of the abdomen. Children under the age of two are thought to be particularly susceptible to the disease.

The symptoms were described as follows: "You can tell when a baby has empacho because it will keep on trying to eat, but will vomit its food as fast as it eats. It also gets colic and cries a lot and may have a little diarrhea and fever. You can diagnose it by feeling the calves of the legs for little bundles or knots along the nerves." The examination for bolitas is performed by rubbing the calf of the leg with a small quantity of lard. If there is empacho, little balls along the nerves can be felt by the examiner. Finding these in one or both legs is thought to establish the diagnosis. If balls are found in the calves, the abdomen is palpated; in empacho a large hard ball in the stomach may be felt.

The disorder is believed to be caused by overeating of certain foods, especially cheese, eggs (in infants only), bananas, and too much soft bread—wheat bread, biscuits, and rolls. Particularly harmful are bananas and *chicharrones* (pork skins fried crisp) if followed by water.

In one reported case there seemed to be some connection between empacho and the "hot and cold" theory. When Rosa's child was diagnosed as suffering from empacho, the child's godparents concluded that the cause of illness was allowing the baby to nurse her bottle too long until the milk got cold. "Her stomach is used to warm milk and the cold milk made her sick."

Paula's treatment for empacho incorporates the use of herbal tea: "You should do this to cure it: you can feel a large hard ball in the stomach. Massage the stomach for a few minutes with a little olive oil. Then immediately have the one with empacho drink a tea, either hot or cold, made of *yerba buena, epazote,* and *manzanilla* [mint, saltwort, and camomile]. These herbs should be boiled for two minutes in one-half cup of water. After the tea, give a good physic; castor oil is best, but milk of magnesia will do. Repeat this for three days, and after that the empacho will be cured."

Barrio people are strong believers in the restorative and prophylactic powers of purges. Men, women, and children are thought to get "dirty stomachs" from time to time. A strong physic is usually administered to each family member two or three times a year to "keep the stomach cleaned out." When a purgative is thought necessary, the patient often drinks a decoction of laxative herbs such as *rosa de castilla,* senna leaves, camomile or cascara bark; castor oil in large quantities is a favorite remedy. Frequent purges are deemed necessary for good digestive function and for preventing empacho.

There is considerable preoccupation with gastrointestinal function. In addition to frequent purging, people also often drink teas of cinnamon bark, wild marjoram, or mint to "soothe the stomach and improve the digestion." Herbs need not be prepared by elaborate methods: garlic shoots, cinnamon bark, coriander, mint, and alfalfa may be chewed in their natural state as a "tonic for the stomach."

Standard Scientific Diseases

A fairly large group of disease conditions recognized by medical personnel are known to the barrio people. Some of these are: *sarampión* (measles), *pulmonía* (pneumonia or bronchitis), *tos ferina* (whooping cough), *asma* (asthma), *tuberculosis, úlcera* (ulcer), *angina* or *mal de garganta* (sore throat), *cáncer* (cancer), *dolor de costado* (side pain, i.e., appendicitis), *resfriado* (head cold), and *cálculos* (stones). The number of scientific medical disorders familiar to the people of Sal si Puedes is constantly increasing as they have more and more contact with members of the English-speaking community and those Spanish-speaking persons in San Jose who are conversant with medical terminology and disease classification.

It should be pointed out, however, that Mexican-Americans who recognize the symptoms of the above diseases and know them by name may often have ideas about etiology that are quite different from the ones accepted by physicians. For example, Concepción reported that her sister's ulcerated throat was the result of the presence in the throat of a foreign object—a small live body, red, looking like a little red rat, the size of the tip of a finger. This object was removed by a curandera. Another example was supplied by Consuela, who attributes cancer and stomach ulcers to the eating of "artificial foods."

Ten patients at the county tuberculosis sanatorium were asked how they came to acquire the disease. Several of the answers revealed that folk beliefs had been used to explain a "standard scientific" disease. For example, Lupe explained: "I got sick after going to a dance. I did a lot of fast dancing, worked up a sweat, and got very hot. Then I drank a bottle of real cold soda water. After that I was never really well again." Lupe's explanation is apparently derived from a local modification of the "hot and cold" theory.

Another tubercular patient attributed her illness to giving a pint of blood at the blood bank for her mother's surgery. Several patients asserted that their tuberculosis was simply a complication of a previous illness. One said, "I had a miscarriage, lost a lot of blood, got weak and run down, and got pneumonia. Then I found out it had gone into TB." Both these explanations illustrate the belief, common in parts of Mexico,[3] that a person must have a large quantity of blood in order to preserve health; if a person loses blood in even small quantities, he may fall ill.

Another cause listed for tuberculosis was preëxisting diabetes: "I think my diabetes brought on the tuberculosis—diabetes is a very dangerous disease; it can cause a lot of other things." Two of the ten patients mentioned malnutrition and exposure to cold and dampness as the cause of their illness. Only one patient, out of the ten questioned, reported that she acquired the disease from contact with another infected person.

Just as folk beliefs may be used to explain the etiology of "scientific" diseases, so folk cures may be prescribed in their treatment. Holy water from the church, for example, is used as a specific for various disorders. Elena reported this case: "When my little boy was born, he had one eye swollen shut for three weeks after the birth. The eye ran all the time. I took him to the doctor, who put some drops in his eye, but that didn't help. Then I rubbed the baby's eyelid with olive oil, but that didn't help either. Finally I took the baby to church and put holy water on his eyelid in the Sign of the Cross, and the eye got well. I guess it was because I had faith in the holy water. My brother's little baby had the same thing when

---

[3] See Beals [3]. Saunders [43] also refers to ideas about blood: "Blood is considered important in the balance of health and disease. . . . Loss of blood for any reason, even in the small amounts necessary for laboratory tests, is thought to have a weakening effect, particularly in males, whose sexual vigor is thereby believed impaire'

he was born. I told my sister-in-law to put holy water on the eye and it would get well. That's what she did, and it did get well."

A patient at the county tuberculosis sanatorium told of another patient, later discharged as cured, who brought with her to the sanatorium a bottle of holy water. "Every morning she took a little sip of it. I think it helped her, because she was real sick when she came in, and she got well and left the hospital in three months. Most people who are that sick stay a lot longer."

Two aspects of Anglo folk curing have been widely adopted in the treatment of "scientific" syndromes for which Mexican folk medicine has no prescriptions. One of these is the use of patent medicines and tonics which can be bought at all local drugstores. The other is the reliance by some Protestant groups on various forms of faith healing (see chap. 5).

Faith is, of course, an important element in all curing. The mother who used holy water on her baby's eye showed her awareness of this fact: "Maybe it was because I had faith in the holy water." An old grandmother who lives in the barrio uses herbs, massage, and magical spells to cure many of her neighbors. However, she does not prescribe for her own grandchildren; she observed that "you have to have faith in the treatment. My grandchildren are used to the doctor and his medicines. Why should I make them take my medicines instead? If they don't have faith in the remedios, maybe they won't work."

Patent medicines, especially tonics, "cold medicine," cough syrups, and laxatives, are very popular in Sal si Puedes. Salves and liniments, merthiolate, and alcohol are used freely on rashes, bruises, cuts, and all sore or aching parts of the body. Vitamin preparations are growing in popularity, but their purpose and value are not always clearly understood. For example, Juan started taking vitamin pills for "stomach trouble": "I had a rotten taste in my mouth and vomited a lot. I got pretty weak, but then I heard about vitamins and started taking six pills every day. I seem to be better now." Consuela reported that she had an operation for cancer five years ago: "The doctor removed all my organs that time. Then they did another operation a few months later. For four years after that they made me come to the hospital every few months for check-ups. But about a year ago I stopped going there because they never found anything wrong with me and never gave me any treatments.

I haven't been back for a year, but I'm taking vitamin tonic now and I don't need to go to the doctor any more."

Consuela apparently expected, when she went to the doctor for check-ups, to be told something new or to be given some medicine —something positive to show her that she needed medical care. The mere fact that the doctor found her in good health, with no further evidence of cancer, was not enough. The notion of the value of a medical check-up was not clear to her and had no significance.

MEDICAL RELATIONS IN SAL SI PUEDES

The social reactions of Mexican-Americans to disease often differ significantly from those of Anglos. For example, how is the decision reached that a person is ill enough to require medical treatment? Who makes such decisions? How is a sick person supposed to behave? Is he exempt from ordinary tasks? Do others blame him for his illness? Does he blame himself? What are his relatives expected to do? What sort of behavior is expected of a doctor or a nurse? All in all, what happens in a barrio when one of its members falls ill?

THE SEQUENCE OF MEDICAL EVENTS

There is no single picture which can portray adequately all the human interrelationships brought into play by illness in Sal si Puedes. The things that happen as a result of sickness vary greatly from one patient to another and from one family to another. Some of the attitudes, behaviors, and procedures frequently encountered, however, are illustrated in the following examples.

What Happened When Rosa Got Sick.—During the Christmas season of 1954, the women of the Sociedad Guadalupana (Altar Society) celebrated Las Posadas. On the nine nights before Christmas Day, processions were formed to carry the images of Mary and Joseph through the streets of the barrio. The faithful participants, among them Rosa, braved icy winds and cold drizzling rain for three nights to celebrate Christmas in the traditional way of the Mexican people. On the fourth night of Las Posadas, Rosa caught a severe cold. The next day she took some aspirin, made a cough syrup of honey and lemon juice, and stayed at home. When night came, however, she did not feel justified in staying at home because the Posadas procession was to originate at the home of her comadre. She again went out to walk through the winter rain in the procession. Three days before Christmas Rosa began to think that what she had considered a common cold was actually something more serious: she had a high fever, headache, a bad cough, and pains in her chest. That night, however, she went out to the Posadas once more. When she returned home, she felt much worse. Her husband became concerned about her high fever and suggested that perhaps she should see a doctor. She assured him that she would be all right in a few days, took some aspirin, and went to bed. The following morning she felt much worse; she had such acute chest pains that she called one of her comadres and her sister, who stayed with her throughout the day. Her comadre made Rosa a pot of orégano tea, and she drank several cups of the hot liquid. By evening her chest pain was more severe, and she was unable to get out of bed. She continued to take aspirin and use Vicks VapoRub on her chest, but was unable to sleep during the night.

The next morning, Christmas Eve, Rosa's chest pains had become so severe that her breathing was labored; she realized that she was extremely ill and would have to consult a doctor. However, she did not suggest seeing a doctor and did not ask anyone to call a doctor for her. She asked her husband to rub her chest with a liniment containing camphor, but that treatment did not relieve her pain. About four hours later, Rosa's husband and sister had a family conference and decided that it was necessary to call a doctor. They were unable to locate a physician who would make a house call on Christmas Eve, so they took her to a doctor's office for treatment.

The doctor told her that she had lobar pneumonia and should be hospitalized. The family had no funds for hospitalization and were not eligible for county hospital service. Rosa asked that she be treated at home if possible. The doctor was sympathetic with Rosa's desire to remain with her family during the Christmas season and to avoid the expense of hospitalization; he discussed the matter with Rosa's husband and sister and finally agreed that she could be treated at home provided she stay in bed for at least two weeks with no unnecessary activity. The doctor administered a shot of penicillin, explained to Rosa's sister how to contrive a vaporizer tent of bedsheets, and arranged to visit the patient at home the following day.

Rosa and her family went home, and for the following week her sister, sister-in-law, and two comadres took turns staying with her, preparing meals for the family, and doing the housework. The patient recovered sufficiently within ten days to resume some of her household duties. She and her family were pleased with her treatment and her recovery. She commented later, "That doctor was just fine. He let me stay at home and he didn't scold me for getting sick—he just said that if I ever got that sick again I should try to see him a little earlier. The next time I get pains like that in my chest I won't wait so long."

What Happened When Lupita Got Sick.—When Manuela's small daughter, Lupita, was an infant, she suffered a gastrointestinal disorder. The events of the illness were as follows.

First day: The child cried a great deal and took less than her accustomed quantity of formula.

Second through fourth days: Lupita continued to cry much more than usual, rejected several of her feedings, and slept for only short periods of time, crying the remainder of the night.

Fifth day: The baby began to have liquid stools and continued to cry almost continuously. Her mother discovered that her abdomen was slightly distended and took the child to be examined by the baby's baptismal godmother. The madrina discovered that the child was cutting an upper tooth and attributed the child's condition to teething. She dipped a small piece of rag in some whiskey and the child was allowed to chew this. The mother thought she saw a little improvement in Lupita's condition, but the child continued to have diarrhea and cried intermittently throughout the night.

Sixth through eighth days: Lupita developed a high fever, had persistent diarrhea, and began vomiting; she took none of her formula.

Ninth day: The symptoms continued, and the child still did not eat. Manuela became alarmed and once more contacted her comadre for advice. Arrangements were made to take the child the following day to the comadre's mother-in-law, a curandera in a neighboring barrio.

Tenth day: The infant was examined by the curandera, who made a diagnosis of empacho. The child's back and legs were rubbed with warm olive oil and then massaged for some time. She was then given a small dose of powdered chalk.

Eleventh day: There was no improvement in the child's symptoms so Manuela took her back for a second treatment.

Twelfth day: Lupita continued to have a high fever, vomiting, and diarrhea; refused all feedings; and cried incessantly. Manuela was visited that day by her sister-in-law, a practical nurse, who advised her to take the baby to a doctor without delay. The child was examined and treated by a pediatrician that afternoon. An oral antibiotic was administered and continued for two days.

Thirteenth day: The child's fever abated and other symptoms were much improved. She began to take some water and formula again.

Fourteenth day: Lupita had no symptoms, stopped crying, and had apparently recovered.

Manuela, in recounting the story of the child's illness some time later, recalled it in this way: "When Lupita was less than a year old, she got empacho. She was pretty sick. I took her to a curandera who is the mother of Lupita's godfather. She rubbed the baby with oil and gave her some white medicine. She did that for two days and then the baby got well." In retrospect, Manuela attributed the child's cure not to the pediatrician's medicine (which she had forgotten completely) but to the treatment given by the curandera.

What Happened When Marta Got Sick.—In the fall of 1955, Marta, a thirty-eight-year-old housewife, began to feel ill. Although she was in the eighth month of her seventh pregnancy, Marta had not yet been to a doctor for prenatal care. The first months of her pregnancy had been relatively uneventful, but during the later months she began to have severe upper abdominal pain, with vomiting and diarrhea after meals. Her discomfort was so intense that she was unable to sleep more than two or three hours each night.

Marta was reasonably sure that she was suffering from gallbladder disease. (Following an attack and hospitalization four years previously, that diagnosis had been made.) In spite of acute discomfort, however, she did not consult a doctor.

Marta had not always been so reluctant to seek medical treatment; her first five babies had been delivered in county hospitals in California. During her fifth pregnancy, however, she had had an unpleasant experience which had altered her attitude toward hospital care. Marta was an obese woman and had steadily gained weight during her childbearing years. She considered this a normal concomitant of maternity. "Almost everybody I know gets fat when they have a lot of babies," she observed. Therefore Marta was totally unprepared for criticism when she reported to the county hospital for prenatal care and was informed that she was disgracefully fat: "They really bawled me out. One nurse said I was as big as a cow and should be ashamed of myself. I was so mad and so embarrassed that I could have died!"

After Marta's fifth delivery, she had suffered her first attack of cholecystitis and had been hospitalized. She had been quite ill and very frightened during that time. "They kept me there for two weeks and wouldn't let me eat anything or have any water—just ice and water in my veins. I don't care if I am fat; it's dangerous to go so long without food. I might have died!" On the basis of her previous experience, Marta assumed that the doctors and nurses at the hospital were maliciously withholding food from her because of her obesity. She had other complaints about her hospital care: "They wouldn't even let me go to the bathroom; I had to use a bedpan and the nurses were always leaving me uncovered there without my clothes on. I couldn't stand that. And they wouldn't let me see my kids."

Marta was particularly disturbed about her children because during her hospital stay her oldest son was involved in a theft and was placed in juvenile hall. Marta contended that if she had not been absent from home for so long, this misfortune would not have occurred.

The following year Marta's feeling of antagonism toward medical workers was intensified. She reported: "When Ricky [her fifth child] was a baby, the district nurse used to come around to see him. She told me that he was old enough to be walking, and that he couldn't walk yet because he was too fat. The nurse said to stop giving him milk and just give him table food. But Ricky kept on getting fatter anyway. Then the nurse told me to take the baby off table food, too. That woman was crazy if she thought I was going to starve my boy to death—he had to eat *something!* Besides, when a child gets ready to walk, he will walk. My other kids had all been fat, too, and they had all learned how to walk by themselves, without the nurse to show them how."

Marta may have misunderstood the district nurse and thought that she was advising complete withdrawal of food from the baby. On the other hand, Marta's version of the incident may have been a contrived story depicting her dislike of the nurse's "interfering" with her child's "normal" growth and development. In any event, this encounter with the district nurse did not improve Marta's opinion of medical personnel.

The year after her hospitalization Marta's husband got a steady job, and through his employer the family acquired hospitalization benefits. This coverage, however, was confined to hospital care and did not include physician's fees, office visits, or out-patient care. The policy did, however, pay the cost of maternity care up to $50. Because of their health-plan coverage, Marta's family was no longer eligible for care at the county hospital. With so many children in the family it became difficult to pay for the medical care which the family required. They were able to obtain better housing and supply their children with a more adequate diet than before, but family income could not be stretched to include the cost of private medical care other than emergency treatments.

In 1952 Marta once again became pregnant. She telephoned the county hospital to ascertain if arrangements could be made for the hospital to accept the $50 health-plan benefits as full payment for her forthcoming delivery. Marta's command of English was rather poor, and she was unable to make herself understood to the Anglo social worker who received her call. When, reportedly, the social worker simply hung up the telephone in the middle of Marta's explanation, Marta felt deeply offended. She became even more convinced that medical workers were discourteous, insulting, rude, and perhaps malicious. She made no further attempts to get information about obstetrical care. When the time came for Marta to deliver her sixth child, she made no effort to go to a hospital or call in a physician; with the assistance of her husband and a neighbor who "had helped with babies in Mexico," she had the baby at home.

When she got sick in 1955, she thought about going to a doctor. A comadre of hers recommended a local private physician. When one of her children needed medical care, Marta took the child to the recommended doctor for treatment. She intended, after the child was treated, to ask the doctor about acting as her obstetrician. However, in the course of his examination of the child, he asked Marta how many children she had. When she explained that she was expecting her seventh baby, the doctor exclaimed, "Seven children! That's too much family; nobody should have that many kids." Marta felt once again that she was being unduly criticized and hastily withdrew from the doctor's office without mentioning maternity care.

Marta was faced with a serious conflict. She described her problems at that time: "I know I'm pretty sick with my gall bladder. I'm supposed to be on a diet—just plain vegetables, lean meat, and cottage cheese, but I can't stay on a diet like that because we don't have the money to buy special foods. I'm afraid to go to a doctor because I'm pretty sure he would put me in the hospital, and I don't think I could stand that again. Besides, we don't have the money for it—our hospital policy won't pay much of the bill. Another thing—one of my boys is on probation now with the juvenile police, and another one keeps trying to quit school. I know if he does that, he'll start running around with bad company and get in trouble. I've got to stay home to keep the kids in school—that's the important thing."

Marta also felt that other members of the family needed medical attention more than she did. "The baby has a bad cold and has been sickly for a couple of months. The next to the youngest needs to have six teeth fixed by the dentist. Then I'm worried about my oldest girl, too. I'm afraid she might have TB or rheumatic fever because she has colds all the time and a cough."

Marta was unable to make a decision about her own illness. She continued to feel progressively worse. Often she would waken during the night with vomiting and diarrhea. When this happened, her husband would make her a tea of cinnamon bark to "settle her stomach."

Marta's medical conflict began to be resolved just one month before her expected delivery date. In response to a request from the school nurse, she was present while her daughter was examined by the school physician. After the child was examined, the doctor inquired in a casual and friendly way about Marta's plans for the new baby. Marta replied that she had not yet seen a doctor and that she had delivered her last child at home by herself. The physician made no comment about Marta's unsupervised delivery, but asked her if she would prefer having the baby in a hospital where she could have better care. After Marta explained her financial situation, the school physician made a telephone call and arranged for her to be seen in a local hospital on a part-pay basis. The school doctor and nurse spent an extra half-hour talking with Marta about her problem. Their patience and courtesy impressed Marta, and she began to think that perhaps she should, after all, go to the hospital.

She immediately went to visit one of her comadres to discuss the problem. It was decided that Marta should follow the doctor's suggestion, and a telephone call was made to the hospital to arrange an appointment. Marta's conference with her comadre lent her the reassurance she needed to carry out the plan suggested by the school physician.

When Marta's husband came home from work that night, she told him of her plan and got his approval. She asked an English-speaking friend to accompany her to the hospital, thus acquiring both transportation and an interpreter in case she should have difficulty communicating with the hospital personnel.

Marta's first interview was with the hospital social worker. He was courteous and pleasant, putting Marta at ease and preparing her for her following visit to the clinic. In the clinic, Marta was fortunate in having a courteous reception. She later related some of her experiences there: "When I went in for my examination, I was really scared—I thought they would be really mean to me. I was expecting a lot of touble when the nurse asked me how many times I had been pregnant and I told her seven times. But she just smiled and said, 'That's a nice family.' Then when they weighed me and I was so fat, I thought, 'Now I'm going to get it!'; but the nurse said she had been pregnant herself and knew how hard it was to stay on a diet. The doctor told me the same thing, but he did explain to me that I shouldn't gain any more weight because I might have a hard time delivering the baby." Marta was immensely relieved by these pleasant encounters. On her way home she stopped at a grocery store and bought some cottage cheese for her diet.

Marta's seventh child was delivered safely; her neighbors and comadres cared for her other children during her hospitalization; her husband kept the older boys out of trouble; and, because of the efforts of interested medical workers, the family was saved from grave financial strain.

As a result of Marta's pleasant medical experiences, her attitude toward medical workers was greatly modified. When the district nurse next came to visit her, Marta inquired about the local child-health conference clinic. She discovered that her grandchildren were eligible for that service and immediately telephoned her married daughter and literally ordered her to take the children to the clinic the following week. As she hung up the telephone, Marta smiled and explained to the nurse: "My daughter is pretty young and doesn't know about these things. She doesn't like doctors much and I'm pretty sure the kids don't have their shots yet."

What Happened When Antonio Got Sick.—In the winter of 1954, Antonio had a job pruning fruit trees. Day after day he worked in the winter cold, often drenched by sudden showers of rain. Antonio felt that he was a fortunate man to have work during the rainy season when so many of his neighbors were without jobs. In January of 1955, he caught a bad cold: he had pain in his chest and fever at night. His wife tried to persuade him to stay home from work for a few days, but he insisted on working. He was worried about his family and about being able to buy enough food for them and about making the payments on his house. He was afraid that if he failed to go to work he might lose his job. He assured his wife and his friends that he was not very sick.

Antonio also took a certain pride in his stamina. He sometimes remarked that his grandfather had been *puro indio,* "pure-blood Indian," and that everyone knows that Indians are tough and strong.

In spite of his determination to ignore his illness, Antonio's condition became worse. His chest and back pain was severe, and he began to lose weight. His wife, concluding that he had the flu, gave him herbal teas and rubbed his chest with volcanic oil. This treatment did little to help him, and he finally decided to consult a doctor.

Some of Antonio's relatives recommended a certain doctor who advertised his services in the local Spanish-language newspaper. This doctor, a chiropractor, took some X rays of Antonio's back and told him that his symptoms were due to "something wrong with his spine" and recommended a series of back "adjustments." He continued to be treated by the chiropractor for about a month, but when his symptoms persisted he concluded that medical science could not help him.

Antonio spent the next two months at home and grew progressively worse. His relatives and friends tried to persuade him to see another doctor, but he said he had already tried one and was sure he could not be helped. Finally one of his cousins came to visit him and insisted that Antonio accompany him downtown to make a purchase. The cousin drove Antonio directly to the county hospital and, once there, persuaded him to go into the clinic. He was examined and found to have pulmonary tuberculosis. Antonio remained in the county tuberculosis sanatorium for the rest of the year.

At first Antonio was angry with his relatives for having tricked him into getting medical attention; he was worried about his family and what would become of them, and he was uneasy in his new surroundings. "I was pretty scared when I first came to the hospital," he said, "because I wasn't used to being around so many Anglos —I had always been around Mexican people most of the time, and I didn't know how they would treat me here. Now I'm used to it, and it doesn't bother me any more. Now I'm afraid to go home because of what people will say about me. People like to hurt your feelings sometimes, and I'm afraid they will treat me funny, like I was a freak. Once I had some visitors here, and do you know what they said? They told me that they had heard I had TB and they wanted to see me before I died! That sure didn't make me feel any better."

The hospital was a strange and unfamiliar place. Antonio spoke English fairly well, but was always a little afraid that he wouldn't be able to think of the right words when he needed them. At first he had a hard time communicating his needs, but gradually he learned new words for the strange kinds of apparatus that are a part of hospital life. He had the idea that if he was sick enough to be put in a hospital he must be very sick indeed, perhaps fatally ill. Gradually this fear was dispelled, and he began to think in terms of recovery.

One thing that helped Antonio to adjust to hospital life was his contact with other Spanish-speaking patients. Frank, a "veteran" sanatorium patient, explained in Spanish many things which English-speaking nurses and doctors had not made clear. Later, when Antonio himself became familiar with hospital customs and procedures, he was able to help new Mexican-American patients with advice and encouragement. Occasionally he tried to talk to some of the viejitos, the elderly men. "When we get a patient who doesn't speak English," he said, "sometimes I try to explain the treatments to them. It's pretty rough on the old people. They don't have much faith in the doctors or the medicines, and it's hard to make them understand anything about what's going on. Always they are scared and very sad."

Antonio's conversations with other Spanish-speaking patients were sometimes interrupted by hospital personnel: "Some of the nurses get real mad when we speak Spanish to each other; some of them bawl us out every time they hear us speak Spanish and tell us that as long as we are in an American hospital we'll have to speak English."

When Antonio was criticized for speaking his own language to fellow patients, he sometimes felt that he was being discriminated against because of his Mexican background. For a day or two after such criticism, he tended to regard any kind of differential treatment as an indication of anti-Mexican prejudice: "Jerry [an Anglo patient] asked for a new mattress for his bed and got it right away even though his old one was all right; but an old Mexican man on our ward really needed a new one because his sagged down in the middle, but the nurse wouldn't give him one." Trivial differences which Antonio might otherwise have recognized as coincidental or inevitable took on a sinister meaning to him on the days when he was told, "This is an American hospital—no Spanish allowed!" In his mind this came to mean, "This is an American hospital—no Mexicans wanted—Mexicans don't belong!"

All during his hospitalization Antonio's family was uppermost in his thoughts. He worried about his wife: would she be faithful to him or would she leave him for another man who was not sick, one who could work hard and make a good living? He worried about his children: who would keep his sons out of trouble and prevent their "keeping bad company" with the tough kids in the barrio? Who would see to it that men did not take advantage of his daughters? Antonio remembered other families he had known and things that had happened when fathers could not provide for their children: "Sometimes boys drop out of school because they have to help the family; it may be the father's fault. Everything I have is my wife and kids—they come first, but I can't help them right now. A man should take care of his family."

While Antonio was hospitalized his wife and children were given a small monthly allowance through the state aid to needy children program. But Antonio began to worry about what would happen when he was discharged from the hospital. While he was a sanatorium patient, he had been convinced that he could not return to strenuous work if he was to avoid a relapse. Antonio's fellow patient, Frank, for example, was in the sanatorium for the second time: "Frank was cured once, but they stopped his family's money from the government, and he had to go back to work too soon —the night shift at the cannery. Man, that night shift can get pretty rough!"

When Antonio was discharged from the sanatorium late in 1955, his economic problems were overwhelming. He was torn between the desire to provide for his family and the sure knowledge that if he returned to agricultural labor, he would likely have to return to the hospital. After a period of vacillation, he agreed that his wife should get a job as a domestic worker. His brother supplied him with small gifts of money from time to time and the family was thus able to survive. Antonio continued to go to the county hospital out-patient clinic for periodic treatments, made some repairs on his house, rested as much as he could, and waited for the day when he would be well again. "My grandfather was *puro indio*," he said, "and everybody knows that Indians are very patient people."

ANALYSIS OF MEDICAL RELATIONS IN SAL SI PUEDES

The preceding four episodes illustrate some common reactions to sickness. Each case of illness presents singular features, but nearly all exhibit certain recurrent social patterns. The following pages discuss some of the common behavior patterns associated with illness in Sal si Puedes.

Individual Reactions to Illness

Most residents of Sal si Puedes regard illness as a distinctly unpleasant state. In addition to the actual physical pain and suffering involved, "being sick" deprives the patient of certain social privileges which he would otherwise enjoy. Barrio people sometimes fear that if they become ill their family and friends will somehow lose respect for them. As Antonio said, "Now I'm afraid to go home [from the hospital] because of what people will say about me." Antonio feared social disapproval—he wanted his social group to view him as a "whole man," a fully functioning member of society and thus entitled to respect and admiration.

Because Sal si Puedes people do not want to be thought "different" or "inferior," they do not readily succumb to illness. Life as they see it is full of countless pains and traumas. Hunger, grief, cold, fear, pain—these things are all a part of life and should be borne with courage and dignity. When Rosa and Antonio began to feel sick, they each made an effort to continue regular activities and duties as long as possible. They would have regarded "giving in" to illness with the first appearance of symptoms as an admission of weakness or lack of stamina. Rosa, with lobar pneumonia, continued to participate in the Posadas—it was her responsibility. Antonio, with early symptoms of tuberculosis, worked on in the fruit orchards during winter storms; he took pride in his strength and in his ability to carry on in the face of infirmity.

Men of the barrio tend to be particularly spartan in their attitudes toward illness. A man who admits to illness is not *macho* (tough and rugged).[4] He feels, as do many Anglos, that sickliness reflects moral weakness. Relatives and friends commend him for endurance and sometimes criticize him when he yields to an infirmity before it becomes acute. Pete's wife related proudly, "Once Pete had chills and fever for four days and nights; he couldn't sleep, but he worked every day just the same." Pete accepted this comment as praise; he was visibly proud of his endurance record.

Women who have relatives or comadres living close by can ordinarily be relieved of more duties during illness than can men. A man cannot send a substitute to his place of employment. Unless he is one of the few barrio men with steady jobs and sick leave, his earnings stop when he falls ill. Housework, however, can usually be taken over by someone else for a day or two without seriously inconveniencing other family members. For women who work out-

---

[4] Beals [4] has commented on the Mexican-American pattern of *machismo*, or rugged masculinity: "Older boys have a strong urge to express their masculinity. They feel they must be *muy hombre* (much the man)."

side the home, illness must be ignored if possible, for their earnings are usually of paramount importance. During the strawberry harvest in 1955, Mercedes began to suffer from acute asthma. When she consulted a doctor, he told her that she was allergic to an insecticide spray used on the berry plants, and advised her to stop work altogether. Mercedes stayed at home one day and then went back to the strawberry patch. "Sure, I have a hard time with the asthma," she explained, "but if I don't work now I'll have a worse time next winter when there's no money for food."

The practice of ignoring illness is not expected of pregnant women, however. Pregnancy is not considered an illness, but barrio people do regard the state as a "delicate" one. Women are free to restrict their activities at that time in order to assure a safe delivery of a healthy child.

Children are less frequently expected to ignore physical symptoms. The younger the child the less stoic he is expected to be. Some of the adult emphasis on strength and stamina, however, carries over into attitudes toward sick children. Youngsters may be sent to school with colds, tonsillitis, skin eruptions, or ear infections. Since they "don't seem very sick," they are expected to carry on normal activities until disease becomes incapacitating. Danny, aged fifteen, had cavities in several of his teeth. His parents had many financial worries at that time and felt that they could not afford dental care for him. He began to have toothaches and complained to his mother who gave him a little whiskey to drink. As long as this medication controlled the pain somewhat, Danny was sent to school as usual. "He's a pretty big boy," his mother commented, "and I guess he can stand it a little longer." Danny was finally taken to a dentist only when toothache kept him awake and pacing the floor at night.

A second aspect of individual reaction is the placement of blame for illness. Generally the sick person is not held responsible for becoming ill. In Anglo groups one often hears these remarks: "I got sick because I didn't take care of myself"; "I'm sorry that I got sick." These ideas, common in the lives of many Americans, reflect a sense of guilt on the part of the sick person. He is often apologetic for an illness, perhaps because others—his family, his friends, or his doctor—remind him that he neglected to take steps to avoid disease: "Why didn't you take care of yourself?"

With a wider public awareness of contagion, preventive medicine, and hygiene, there is a tendency to place blame for illness on the patient or those responsible for his welfare. In some segments of Anglo society a patient (or his parents if the patient is a sick child) is expected to accept the responsibility for disease and somehow to atone for his misdemeanor by feeling guilty, by accepting even vitriolic criticism, by offering apologies, and by promising to "repent and sin no more." Thus a doctor at the county hospital scolded the father of a sick child: "You're not a very good father to allow your child to get in this condition." When the father showed no sign of accepting responsibility for his son's ailment, the doctor assumed that the man was either stupid or unconcerned with the child's welfare.

Among the Spanish-speaking folk of Sal si Puedes, the patient is regarded as a passive and innocent victim of malevolent forces in his environment. These forces may be witches, evil spirits, the consequences of poverty, or virulent bacteria which invade his body. The scapegoat may be a visiting social worker who unwittingly "cast the evil eye." It may be a member of the sick man's social group who "made him sick" by frightening him, making him angry, or otherwise upsetting him emotionally. Blame may be projected to the demands of life in urban America.

Mexican folk concepts of disease are based in part on the notion that people can be victimized by the careless or malicious behavior of others. Thus illness is sometimes an effective tool of social control. This topic is reviewed below in the discussion of social functions of illness.

There is one idea about disease which places responsibility on the patient. Teresa remarked, "Sometimes people can get sick as a punishment for their sins. If you know you have done something bad but you don't go to confession and get God to forgive you, this stays on your mind and you get worried and even sick. If people would confess their sins and pray, they would get well a lot faster." Although this view of sickness as a punishment for wrongdoing is present in the barrio, it is not a central theme in attitudes toward disease. The concept is always connected with the idea of moral offense and is rarely extended into the nonreligious facets of life. The patient is blamed not for becoming ill but for failing to perform the religious obligation of confession.

In summary, barrio people do not like to admit an illness lest their associates think them weak or lacking in stamina. They try to "be strong" and often refuse to accept the fact that they are sick until they become acutely ill. Once the idea of illness has been accepted, however, a patient rarely thinks of blaming himself for the disorder. He has done what he could to withstand disease. He is not responsible for getting sick; illness just happens to people.

Social Functions of Illness

Illness among the Mexican-American people of Sal si Puedes has both negative and positive results. For most people the negative results greatly outweigh the positive ones. They view illness as a state of physical and emotional discomfort, costly in time and money, sometimes threatening to social relationships, uncertain in duration and intensity, and possibly debilitating or even fatal in consequence. Barrio people realize, however, that some illness of a milder sort carries with it certain incidental advantages. A factory worker observed, "I felt pretty bad when I had the flu, but at least I got a chance to rest for a few days." Illness performs functions far more significant than this, however; it sometimes plays a vital role in stabilizing social relations within the community.

The following six case studies illustrate the functions of illness.

First, illness may serve to publicize and punish social offenses. When someone gets sick, his ailment may be interpreted by the community as the natural result of conflict with another member of his social group. Sickness focuses attention on the person or persons who have "mistreated" him; group disapproval and disciplinary action may be brought to bear on those judged responsible for his illness. This function of illness is illustrated by the following case.

Case 1.—A young woman expecting her first child became angry with her husband one night when he came home drunk. She scolded him thoroughly for this, whereupon he beat her and put her out of the house in the rain. She walked to her mother's house, some blocks away, where she related her trying experience. Her relatives immediately took her to a curandera for treatment for fear that her unborn child would suffer later from susto, or "fright."

This young wife felt that she had been badly abused by her husband. Ordinarily she would not have been thought justified under the circumstances in openly condemning her husband for beating her. After all, she had scolded him and insulted him for getting drunk with his friends—a type of entertainment regarded by many barrio men as their prerogative. Because his wife was pregnant, however, she had recourse to a folk-defined disease, susto, and she thus acquired the status of a patient. There was a possibility that her baby might be born with susto as a result of the "fright" she had received; thus she gained the sympathy and support of her entire social circle. Soon the news of her unfortunate experience spread through the barrio, and open criticism was directed against the un- feeling husband who had threatened the life of his unborn child. He was finally persuaded of the error of his ways; he made the necessary apologies and promises, and the couple was happily re- united.

Illness has a second important social function: it provides escape from social disapproval by affording a rationale for otherwise un- sanctioned behavior. This is best illustrated by the following case.

Case 2.—A young man jilted his fiancée. About a week later, he became ill. The patient discussed his symptoms with his brother, and the conclusion was reached that the young man was *embrujado,* bewitched; the jilted girl, it was decided, had cast a spell on him and caused him to get sick. Since his symptoms persisted, the patient was finally seen by a doctor, who diagnosed his illness as influenza. The medical diagnosis in no way changed the attitudes of the patient or his family about the ultimate cause of the disorder— whatever the disease might be, it was surely the result of malevolent witchcraft.

This illness, as perceived by the patient and his family, resulted from witchcraft, which in turn was induced by a social offense on the part of the patient. In a sense the illness was his punishment for breach of contract. Since, however, it was decided that the jilted girl either was a witch herself or had hired someone else to cast an evil spell, the illness was interpreted as proof of the girl's wicked and malicious nature. The patient's conscience was thus cleared of guilt for rejecting her. He no longer owed her anything —he was, by his illness, relieved of any further social obligation. The illness of the reluctant bridegroom thus served to alter public opinion. He was no longer condemned for jilting his fiancée—after all, a man cannot be expected to marry a woman who might be a malevolent witch.

The following case illustrates another way in which illness serves to offset social disapproval. It differs from case 2 only in terms of time sequence. In case 2 the illness followed a breach of conduct and afforded a rationalization for the offense. In the following case the patient was faced with obligations which she did not welcome. She became ill and her illness was accepted as sufficient cause for subsequent exemption from her normal social responsibilities. Behavior which would have been severely criticized in a healthy person was permitted and even encouraged in a sick one.

Case 3.—A couple with six children found themselves faced with acute financial problems as a result of a prolonged visit by the husband's brother, his wife, and their five children. The visiting brother had come to San Jose to seek work, but had not found a job after three weeks. Both families—fifteen persons in all—were living in a three-room house and trying to subsist on the wages of one common laborer. Their debt at the grocery store grew larger and larger, and finally the grocer would no longer extend them credit.

The woman of the house felt obliged to provide food and shelter for her needy relatives; at the same time, she feared that as a result of her hospitality her own children would have to go hungry. She began to suffer from shortness of breath, sweating, and rapid pulse. She discussed her symptoms with her sister and two of her comadres, who assured her that she was suffering from susto, or "fright." A neighborhood curandera was called in to diagnose and treat her for this disorder. When it was established that the woman was asustada, "frightened," relatives and comadres insisted that she was ill, and should not have the responsibility of cooking for her brother-in-law's family. The visitors were encouraged to move on to another area where jobs were more plentiful.

Illness in this case served to excuse the patient from social responsibility. This woman could not openly refuse to sacrifice the comfort of her own children in order to provide for destitute relatives. She would have been condemned as a selfish and unfeeling woman who cared nothing about her husband's family. However, when financial worries became acute, she began to have shortness of breath and other symptoms of anxiety. The symptoms were attributed to susto, a folk disease. Her illness was recognized, and her intimates insisted on a change to relieve her of extra responsibility. When the change was made, her anxiety was relieved and her symptoms disappeared. Her rapid recovery was attributed to the excellence of the cure performed by the local curandera.

Illness has a third important function. It is a means of dramatizing to others the evil consequences of cultural change and of defending the "old ways"—Mexican customs and traditions which are under constant attack in the United States. This is done by attributing disease to the demands of Anglo society or to the ways of American life which are uncongenial to the patient. Several cases were observed.

Case 4.—A grandmother, born and reared in Mexico, claimed that she has suffered from "stomach trouble" since moving to the United States. This, she said, is due to the "artificial" food which she is forced to eat in this country.

A higher incidence of gastrointestinal upsets, whether real or imagined, was taken by the patient as evidence that things are somehow better in Mexico. This idea may be related to her feeling that she was happier in Mexico and felt more secure, more in tune with life there. Here she apparently feels that she is in an "artificial" environment in which she is unhappy and resentful. Illness is perhaps her symbolic verbalization of nostalgia for home and antagonism toward the United States. To her American-born children and grandchildren she dramatizes her dissatisfaction with life in the United States. She tells them, implicitly, "I was healthy and happy in Mexico, but this place is making me sick."

Case 5.—A middle-aged American-born woman related that she has chronic poor health. Whereas her mother bore many children, never saw a doctor, yet lived to be more than ninety years old, the patient reported that she herself has had an abdominal operation and was able to conceive only one child. The Mexican people in California, she said, generally suffer poor health because of a change in diet. Because of the rapid pace at which people now must live, the women are unable to cook food properly. Eating semiraw food naturally makes people sick, she said.

This woman moved with her husband and other relatives from a small ranch in Arizona to the urban San Jose area where her husband is a construction worker. A required change in time orientation, with regular hours to keep and a time clock to punch, is a new situation for her. She relates her poor health to the rapid pace of her new life.

In the following example of illness as a form of resistance to culture change, the patient attributed her illness to the type of medical treatment she had received for a previous disorder.

Case 6.—An elderly woman was admitted, against her wishes, as a patient in a San Jose hospital. When the acute phase of her illness was past, she was given "bathroom privileges"; that is, the nurse came into her room and insisted that she get up and take a shower. The patient was not accustomed to showers every day—she ordinarily took tub baths at less frequent intervals. She objected to this order, but her objections were ignored, and she was forced to follow the nurse's instructions. Coming back from the shower, she had an attack which she identified as mal aire, "bad air." She had her relatives bring her some herbs marinated in oil for massage of the affected area.

This patient suffered an attack of a folk-defined disorder that she considered the result of hospital treatment of which she disapproved. If she had been left at home or if her judgment had been followed, she believed, this would not have happened. The illness gained her the sympathy of family members and caused them to blame and mistrust the hospital workers whose ignorance and carelessness had "brought on the attack." The patient, at the insistence of her relatives, was prematurely discharged from the hospital and taken home where she could receive "proper care."

It should be emphasized that not every case of sickness among barrio people results in improved social relations. Many illnesses are trying periods of social crisis for the patient and his family; indeed, previously harmonious family life may be disrupted through worry, financial strain, separation of the patient in a hospital, social stigma, or other consequences of disease.

The point illustrated in the six cases above is that some illness is interpreted as related to a derangement or imbalance in human relations. In some of these cases "scientific syndromes" such as influenza are attributed to "pathogenic" factors in the patient's social environment. The ailment has positive social function in that it provides a stimulus for the restoration of social equilibrium.

In other cases emotional disturbances produce symptoms which are defined as illnesses of the "folk-disease" type. It is easy to understand why many Mexican-American people cling to folk-disease concepts. Foster [17] has said that "the pervasiveness of folk medicine, its vitality, and its self-sufficiency are noteworthy. It is not just a question of a random collection of old beliefs and superstitions. Folk medicine flourishes today because it is a functional part of the people's way of life." In Sal si Puedes, folk interpretation of disease is a dramatic means of "acting out" social disturbances resulting in anger, fear, shame, or anxiety. Thus, through disease an individual can demonstrate vividly to others that "something is wrong" with his social environment and that he needs the assurance and support of family, friends, or community. These disorders furnish the group a rationale for making social adjustments advantageous to the patient and to the community as a whole.

There is a striking parallel between certain Mexican folk diseases and some of the "psychosomatic disorders" which have come to the attention of modern physicians within the past few decades. Modern medicine has recognized the emotional etiology of some diseases only recently. Perhaps in this field at least some of the world's less sophisticated peoples have shown a remarkable precocity.

The Role of the Social Group in Illness

People in Sal si Puedes do not act as isolated individuals in medical situations. In illness as well as in other aspects of life, they are members of a group of relatives and compadres. Individuals are responsible to their group for their behavior and dependent on them for support and social sanction. Medical care involves expenditure of time and energy by the patient's relatives and friends. Money for doctors and medicines comes from the common family purse; many of a sick person's duties are performed during the period of illness by other members of his social group. Illness is not merely a biological disorder of the individual organism—it is a social crisis and period of readjustment for an entire group of people.

It is customary, therefore, for an individual to present his symptoms to his relatives and friends for their appraisal before he takes steps to obtain medical treatment. The patient alone is not authorized to decide whether or not he is ill; even though he himself may be convinced that he is sick enough to warrant special attention, his intimates must still be persuaded of the seriousness of his complaints. In other words, an individual is not socially defined as a sick person until his claim is "validated" by his associates. Only when relatives and friends accept his condition as an illness can he claim exemption from the performance of his normal daily tasks.[5]

In relations with medical personnel, then, a patient is not free to make immediate and conclusive decisions concerning his own health. He is acting not as an individual but as a family member. When the school physician advised Marta to report to a local clinic for prenatal care, Marta was unable to say whether she would or would not go. It was not her decision alone to make. She was obliged first to consult her comadre who would be responsible for her children in case she was hospitalized; she had to confer with her husband who would have to assume full responsibility for the family and who would have to furnish money, medicines, and transportation. Only after her husband and her comadre had said, "Yes, Marta, you are sick and should go to the clinic,"—only then could she speak with authority about her medical plans.

Medical decisions concerning children are also made by the family group and not by a single individual. The story was told of a man who had lived in San Jose only six months when one of his children got sick. The child was taken to a county clinic where the doctor recommended a tonsillectomy. The father refused to agree to the operation at that time, saying that he did not know much about that sort of thing and that he had not heard of its being done in Mexico. The doctor was somewhat annoyed because the father would not immediately accept his verdict and authorize the operation. Some time later, however, the father returned to the clinic and said he would like the operation performed. It was discovered that he had discussed the doctor's advice with a number of relatives and neighbors, who agreed that a tonsillectomy was a common and beneficial operation. The consensus favored the medical recommen-

[5] Parsons [36] discusses the "validation" of illness in our own society: "This exemption requires legitimation by and to the various alters involved and the physician often serves as a court of appeal as well as a direct legitimatizing agency . . . the legitimation of being sick enough to avoid obligations . . . has the social function of protection against 'malingering.'"

dation, and so the cautious but conscientious parent consented to have the surgery done.

The pattern of reserving for the group the right to control the medical treatment of its members is sometimes in conflict with the expectations of Anglo health personnel. In the society to which most American doctors and nurses belong, the concept of individual responsibility and self-determination is a well-developed pattern; in Sal si Puedes, it is almost nonexistent. When a Spanish-speaking person is asked to make an on-the-spot medical decision on his own initiative, he is placed in an embarrassing, impossible situation. Frequently, his only choice is to withhold judgment until he discusses the matter with other family members. But, since most barrio people are extremely courteous and gracious and want to avoid dissension, a patient may seem to agree with whatever plan the doctor or nurse presents. "Yes," he says; "Sí that's fine!" Actually, however, the real decision is made after he returns home and talks with his family. If the group decides to reject the arrangements "approved" by the individual for an operation, a hospital admission, or a laboratory test, appointments may be broken without warning, much to the confusion and exasperation of medical workers.

When Antonio was suffering from tuberculosis, for example, his wife tried in vain to encourage him to see a doctor. When she alone was unable to influence him to go, she called in Antonio's cousin—an older male relative with more status and authority in the family than she had—and between the two of them they tricked Antonio into the plan of action which the family had decided was best.

The authority of the family group also supersedes that of the professional medical workers. Opinions of doctors and nurses certainly influence family decisions, but they are not accepted as absolute fact. The unwillingness of barrio people to look upon members of the medical profession as the final authority in medical matters sometimes leads to conflict and antagonism. This reaction to medical authority is discussed in the following topic on the role of the scientific curer.

When the decision is reached that a person is sick and requires special care and attention, his relatives and compadres cluster around him, take over some or all of his duties in the home and the community, and assume full responsibility for his recovery. The following description by Saunders [43] of the role of the family in illness might well have been written about the barrio of Sal si Puedes.

Good medical care, as defined in the culture of the Spanish-Americans, requires that the patient be treated for almost any condition at home by relatives and friends, who are constantly in attendance and who provide emotional support as well as the technical skills required in treatment. In time of sickness one expects his family to surround and support him, and to supervise closely and critically, if not actually carry on, the treatment process. Members of the family, in turn, feel obligated to remain close to the patient, to take charge of his treatment, and to reassure him as to his place in and importance to the family group.

The history of Rosa's illness illustrates clearly the importance of the family in medical treatment. Her husband, her sister, her sister-in-law, and her two comadres formed a family council which decided that she was ill and was to receive medical care. They administered home remedies and patent medicines; they provided nursing care, constant supervision, entertainment, money, and transportation; they took over Rosa's regular duties of cooking, housekeeping, and laundering; they offered prayers for her and arranged for the priest to visit her. Rosa could perhaps have recovered as well had she been hospitalized and isolated from her social group; she would not, however, have recovered so cheerfully and with such reassurance of her importance in her family circle.

THE ROLE OF THE CURER

The first step in the treatment of illness is the mobilization of the resources of the family group. Those who have had experience with illness and "know about sickness and curing" are called upon to diagnose the trouble and use what curing methods they know to combat the disease. If the disorder cannot be diagnosed by members of the family or if the medicaments they suggest fail to halt the course of the illness, the group calls upon friends and neighbors to suggest other cures.

The choice of a curer depends largely on the past experiences and resulting preferences of the family and friends of the patient. If the family has had good relations in the past with physicians and other medical specialists, the patient may be taken directly to a doctor. More frequently, however, the patient first sees a folk curer or a marginal practitioner (chiropractor, herbalist, or homeopath), and only as a last resort goes to a private physician or a medical agency. One San Jose doctor who has a large Mexican-American practice reported that an estimated 50 per cent of all Spanish-speaking patients he sees have first consulted some other type of curer —a curandera, herbalist, or marginal practitioner. An additional 20 per cent, he estimated, have been treated previously with home remedies by relatives or friends. This physician's practice is not confined to low-income groups; his patients are Mexican-American people from all socioeconomic levels in the San Jose colony. It is safe to assume that in a low-income neighborhood like Sal si Puedes, an even larger proportion of people go to doctors only when all other resources have failed.

Assuming that scientific practitioners have a greater wealth of information and techniques for treating illness than do other curers, there must be other factors which outweigh the doctor's technical competence and favor the selection of folk practitioners.

One factor may be that barrio people have definite ideas about how a medical practitioner should behave; these expectations are based largely on the traditional attitudes and actions of Mexican folk curers. Anglo medical workers often behave quite differently —in ways that seem appropriate to them, but which make Mexican-American patients uncomfortable.

It may be instructive to describe the usual behavior and procedures of folk curers, the kind of professional behavior that barrio people have known all their lives and have come to regard as right and proper.

Folk Curers

Folk curers are not professionals in the sense that they have formal training in the art of medicine or earn their living by their practice. They are members of the community who are regarded as specialists because they have learned more of the popular medical lore of their culture than have other barrio people. Paula, for example, is a curandera who is a resident of the barrio. Her patients are often relatives, compadres, or neighbors whom she has known intimately for years. As a Spanish-speaking person, she uses language which they understand. Her professional vocabulary includes few terms which are unfamiliar to her patients.

When Paula is asked to examine a sick person in the barrio, she is called upon both as a curandera and as a friend. People know that she is one of them and that she really cares what happens to them and has their welfare at heart. She sometimes goes to a patient's home if the illness is acute. More often, patients are brought to her house, and she greets them in her kitchen, which smells faintly of the tools of her trade—mint, rosemary, cinnamon, and coriander. Paula's manner is as warm and friendly as her kitchen-dispensary. She observes the requisite social amenities and always behaves in a manner which her clients regard as courteous. For example, she is always careful to wait for an invitation to enter a house before she goes in. She knows that she is expected to sit down with the family, drink a cup of coffee, and make small talk before getting down to the business at hand. This coffee and conversation is protocol in Sal si Puedes; a courteous and well-bred person does not rush into the middle of things. The talk is of work, weddings, the new teacher at the school, the church bazaar—anything but the sick person waiting to be examined. After a "decent" interval, the illness can be mentioned and the patient seen.

Paula's diagnosis does not require that she take a medical history; she has already gotten a good deal of information about the illness from neighborhood gossip. She makes her diagnosis by looking at the patient's eyes and color, feeling his pulse, or palpating his abdomen or the calves of his legs. The diagnosis is usually one that is familiar to the patient and his family—he is suffering from susto or empacho or bilis, or he has been afflicted with aire or mal ojo.

Therapy too is relatively uncomplicated. Topical treatment may be administered on the spot by Paula herself, or she may give instructions for relatives to perform some treatment at home. If medicine is prescribed, Paula may furnish the ingredients from her herb garden, or the compound may be a simple and inexpensive one available at any pharmacy. Relatives are always welcome to make suggestions or criticisms. Paula never dictates what must be done; she simply advises the patient's family of what she considers appropriate treatment. They are free to accept or reject it without any hard feelings.

Paula charges little or nothing for her services. If she believes that the disorder is one which requires the attention of a doctor, she is quick to recommend one who is *simpático* and not too expensive.

Saunders [43] has said that "folk medicine, like scientific medicine, undoubtedly derives much of its prestige and authority from the fact that the majority of sick persons get well regardless of what is done." Perhaps for this reason, Paula's remedies often work well and she has a grateful and devoted clientele.

Paula's ability to gain and hold the confidence of her neighbors is due in part to the fact that she fulfills cultural expectations of the role of a curer. Another force in her favor is that she practices medicine within the familiar context of folk belief.

Writers who have had first-hand experience with other cultures have emphasized again and again the potency and persistence of popular concepts about sickness and health. Saunders [43] said that "the practices and beliefs themselves are often so deeply rooted in tradition that they seem a part of the natural order of things and are as much taken for granted as the daily rising and setting of the sun." Foster [19] emphasized the importance of folk beliefs in medicine: "People generally have very specific ideas about health and illness, and about disease causation and treatment. Whether these ideas are scientifically based, as we feel ours are, or whether they are based on what we consider superstition, human beings everywhere are emotionally attached to them, and passionately believe they are correct." Simmons [44] reported that "in Chile . . . belief in folk medicine pervades even the most highly urbanized communities and plays a substantial part in determining attitudes toward modern medicine."

Among Spanish-speaking families of Sal si Puedes, too, folk medical beliefs have much the same importance that they have in other cultures. A private physician in San Jose was asked what he told his patients when they asked him about folk disorders such as "evil eye." He replied, "I tell them not to believe that—there's no such thing as evil eye." Yet this same physician estimated that 75 per cent of his Spanish-speaking patients ask him about one or another of the folk diseases. A school nurse in Mayfair reported that 25 per cent or more of Mexican-American parents who come to her office mention voluntarily folk diseases or some kind of folk curing practices.

These estimates indicate that folk belief in the barrio is not a trivial or insignificant element in medical care; it is not merely a remnant of primitive superstition that can be miraculously dispelled by a denial of its existence. On the contrary, folk medical beliefs form a persistent framework into which new learning must be fitted. New ideas which are inconsistent with its pattern are likely to be rejected as false or, if there is strong empirical evidence for new ideas, they may be relegated to a special category of disorders "that doctors know about."

From the point of view of at least half the residents of Sal si Puedes, a doctor or nurse who denies the existence of "evil eye" or other folk syndromes is either a fool or a liar. The people *know* that such illnesses exist, and they defend their knowledge vigorously. They are just as convinced of the existence of "evil eye" and "magical fright" as they are of the existence of poliomyelitis.

Actually there are few laymen in Sal si Puedes or elsewhere in the United States who have seen a laboratory demonstration of the polio virus; nor are laymen generally aware of the kinds of experimental study and research required for scientific proof of a hypothesis. Barrio people do not "know" that a virus causes polio—they have not seen the evidence with their own eyes. They simple *believe* in the polio virus, just as they believe in "evil eye."

Logically, arguments in favor of the existence of these two diseases —polio and "evil eye"—are, in the light of a layman's knowledge, equally strong. For example, barrio people have heard about both diseases all their lives and have seen diagnosed patients with their own eyes. In both diseases the cause is established by observing the effects of exposure on a well person. However, all persons exposed to the "causative" factor do not succumb to either disease; some people are considered more resistant than others. For both diseases there are supposed prophylactic measures (vaccine for polio, charms for "evil eye") and accepted forms of therapy; but prophylaxis does not always prevent the disease nor do "cures" always prevent severe illness or even death. In neither disease does the occurrence of a constant group of symptoms prove to the layman the connection with the supposed etiological factor. In neither disease can the layman be sure that the patient did not have something else and merely recovered spontaneously. He simply accepts the testimony of "experts."

The primary difference between barrio belief in folk diseases and barrio acceptance of "scientific syndromes" is that the latter is shared with many Anglo laymen and medical specialists. Anglos generally agree that there is sufficient evidence for accepting the existence of a polio virus; Paula and her neighbors also believe they have enough evidence to prove the existence of "evil eye." To ask barrio people to trust a doctor who says, "There's no such thing as evil eye" is like asking a mother to continue to take her children to a physician who, when she asks "Could it be polio?" says, "Don't believe that—there's no such thing as polio!"

It is not difficult to understand why Manuela, Lupita's mother, attributed the infant's recovery from empacho not to the pediatrician's medicine but to the treatment given the previous day by a curandera. The baby had empacho and the curing woman treated the child for empacho; the pediatrician gave medicine for another disease. After all, how can a doctor cure something he does not even know about?

Marginal Practitioners

Chiropractors, homeopathic physicians, and herbalists have achieved a considerable popularity and prestige among Sal si Puedes families. One reason for their popularity is advertising; practitioners who utilize the Spanish-language radio and press are especially successful in attracting Mexican-American patients.

A second reason for this popularity is that barrio people are not always able to distinguish between chiropractors and medical doctors. When one patient was asked why she had chosen to consult a chiropractor instead of a medical doctor, she replied, "Oh, I'm pretty sure he was a doctor all right—he had "doctor" written on his door and he had diplomas on his wall." Aside from those patients who see marginal practitioners "by accident," there are many who prefer their services to those of a medical doctor. Some barrio people find that chiropractors and homeopaths more nearly fit their expectations of how a curer should behave: they are sometimes more courteous, show more interest in the patient's personal and family problems, and seldom tell a patient that there is "nothing wrong" with him. Generally, a marginal practitioner seems to have a better "bedside manner"; he appears friendly, courteous, sincere, and sympathetic. Moreover, his fees are likely to be lower than those of a medical doctor, he seldom writes prescriptions for costly medicines, and he rarely advises expensive laboratory tests, operations, or hospitalizations.

Another reason for the popularity of marginal practitioners is the types of therapy they administer. Chiropractic treatments, for example, are consistent with the popular Mexican-American belief that many illnesses can be cured by massage and manipulation of "misplaced organs" or the treatment of "coldness" of body parts with topical heat applications. "Adjustments" of the spine, massage, and treatments with infrared lamps, the chiropractor's stock in trade, are types of therapy which the people know and understand.

Herbalists, too, practice a type of therapy which has meaning for Mexican-Americans. Curing with herbs is an ancient and accepted tradition in virtually all Sal si Puedes families. Some of the Mexican-American people complain that "there aren't any good *yerbalistas* [herbalists] here in San Jose. In Mexico you can always find a good one." There are, however, several Chinese herb specialists in the area, and some of them attract Spanish-speaking patients. One San Jose physician reported that a Mexican-American patient who came to him with advanced pulmonary tuberculosis had been under the care of a Chinese herbalist for three years. The fact that Chinese herbalists use an Oriental rather than a Latin-American pharmacopoeia is of no apparent concern to Spanish-speaking patients. The attitude seems to be that "herbs are good"—their nature and origin is relatively immaterial.

The acceptance of marginal practitioners illustrates a point which has significance for public health workers and other medical personnel: Families sometimes seek medical care from curanderas who are members of their own social group, but they will also utilize the services of a non-Spanish-speaking specialist outside the community who does not speak Spanish if the practitioner fulfills the social role expected of a curer, charges reasonable fees, and shows that he knows and respects the folk beliefs and curing practices which are a part of the medical tradition of the Mexican people.

"Scientific" Practitioners

Observers of medical relations in American society have pointed out conflicts between lay expectations and the roles assigned to practitioners by their professions [15, 30, 35, 53]. Certain aspects of the medical-worker's role as he perceives it are even less congenial to Mexican-Americans than they are to English-speaking laymen. Three principal sources of conflict derive from different attitudes toward:

(1) authority of the physician, (2) the objective approach, and (3) the concept of "efficiency."

In the United States the social role of the "scientific" curer demands that he accept responsibility for the patient's recovery and that he be allowed to meet this responsibility by assuming a great deal of control over the patient's actions. A doctor usually expects that the prestige of his training will cause laymen to accept his judgment and to follow his advice. As a highly trained and skilled technician, he expects recognition as the final authority in medical matters. If patients or their families seem hesitant to acknowledge his authority, he may chide them for their failure to recognize his superior knowledge and skill.

The Spanish-speaking people of Sal si Puedes, as illustrated in their family relationships and their community life, are accustomed to authority and are reluctant to defy it. It may seem strange, then, that they so easily and frequently disregard "doctors' orders." The explanation of this seeming paradox is a simple one: the lines of authority in family and community are clearly defined by tradition, but the curer's role in Mexican-American culture is not an authoritarian one. Curers may advise, but they may not dictate. Medical advice may be followed only if it is sanctioned by the powerful members of the patient's social group. Anglo patients, who are accustomed to looking to the "family doctor" for sage advice in many departments of life, may follow "doctors' orders" to change jobs, move to a different neighborhood, abstain from sexual activity, enroll junior in military school, or learn to play golf. The role of the curer, for Spanish-speaking people, is much more restricted—his job is to consult and advise in medical matters. He may diagnose disease and administer appropriate medications only if the patient and his family believe that his prescriptions are necessary and appropriate. Barrio people regard the "nonmedical" aspects of life—employment, residence, sexual contacts, child rearing, and recreation—as lying completely outside the doctor's province. To them the physician is not a final authority. A practitioner who uses an authoritarian approach may be met with an amused but stubborn resistance on the part of his Mexican-American patients. A continued authoritarian approach, in fact, may drive patients away completely as the following case illustrates.

In the years prior to 1952, Lupe Martinez was a regular visitor at one of Santa Clara County's child-health conferences, to which she brought her children for immunizations and check-ups. In 1952, however, the family moved into the district of a public health nurse whose approach to patients was sometimes aggressive and dictatorial. "Once I missed an appointment at the clinic," Lupe reported. "That nurse was real mean. She told me that she was the nurse and that I'd better get the kids to the clinic next time. Boy, that really burned me up!"

For three years following this encounter, Lupe seldom attended the child-health conference. Two new babies born to the Martinez family failed to receive immunizations. Lupe rarely consulted doctors for her children any longer, but instead began to rely on the folk remedies and advice of her mother, who "knew about herbs and medicines." In 1955 Lupe once again moved, this time to a different nursing district. When the family's medical records came to the attention of the new district nurse, she called on Lupe and attempted to discover the reason for her rejection of the public health facilities. Winning Lupe's confidence was not an easy task —the nurse called at the Martinez home many times before Lupe gave her any information. Finally, during one visit, Lupe told the nurse that she had not been bringing her children to the clinic because "my mother knows how to take care of them when they get sick."

Having an awareness of the importance of family authority in medical care, the nurse encouraged Lupe to tell her about some of the remedies her mother had used. Most of the herbal treatments seemed innocuous, and the nurse told Lupe, "Your mother is a wise woman and gives good advice. She has lived longer than you or I, and you do well to listen to her. When you see her again, will you ask her something for me? Ask her what she thinks about giving the children shots so that they will be protected against whooping cough and other diseases. When I visit you again, I would like to know what she thinks about these shots." Lupe did not wait for the nurse's next home visit—she and Mamacita together bundled up the children and brought them to the child-health conference the following week.

Authoritarianism has an important place in Mexican-American culture, but that place is not in relations with "outsiders" such as medical personnel.

The Objective Approach

As Parsons [36] has pointed out, medical training in the United States teaches physicians that scientific accuracy depends on their "affective neutrality." Doctors must repress subjective reactions to their patients, must refrain from interacting emotionally with them, and must remain "clinical" in their attitudes. It is of some interest that the term "clinical" in modern English usage has come to connote a lack of emotion, a coldly impersonal approach—the antithesis of warmth and friendliness. Experienced physicians, however, learn that "bedside manner" is an asset in their contacts with patients.

The people of Sal si Puedes are frightened by illness, perhaps even more frightened than members of other groups. Good "bedside manner" is especially important in the treatment of Mexican-American patients. They expect a curer to reassure them, to show that he sympathizes with them and cares what happens to them. They reason that if the curer has no interest in his patients, he may not really try to help them; he must be practicing medicine for only one reason —to make money. If the physician's approach is too "clinical," his attitude may be interpreted as one of hostility. A high fee confirms the patient's belief that the doctor "doesn't care what happens to me as long as he gets his money." Fees are usually paid willingly, however, if the patient is sure of the doctor's interest and sincerity.

It seems unlikely that a friendly manner toward patients need impair the physician's objectivity. With the Mexican-American patient, who expects curers to take a personal interest in his infirmity, a little extra show of sympathy, warmth, and reassurance may be a decisive factor in the success or failure of the therapeutic relationship. As Marta said, "I was really surprised at that hospital—everybody was so nice!"

The Concept of "Efficiency"

Scientific practitioners through both training and necessity learn to work quickly and efficiently. As a rule doctors lose little time in their dealings with patients—they try to come directly "to the point" and to avoid lengthy discussions with the patient or his relatives. Of course, the amount of time doctors spend with individual patients depends on several factors: the physician's patient load, the complexity or seriousness of the case, the number of hours the doctor is willing to work each day, and the overt time demands of the patient himself. However, most physicians work against time—their schedules are full and their waiting rooms crowded.

San Jose doctors seldom make home calls except to see non-ambulatory patients. Some insist on seeing patients in their offices because they believe they can treat patients more rapidly and more effectively in their own examining rooms where they have access to a greater range of diagnostic tools and the assistance of their office personnel.

Sal si Puedes people prefer to have a doctor examine a sick person at home, but they are not averse to taking a patient to the curer. However, they are often unprepared for the doctor's hurried examination and abrupt dismissal. One of the more frequent complaints heard from Spanish-speaking people is, "The doctor didn't *do* anything—he just saw me for a couple of minutes and gave me some pills." Folk curers, on the other hand, usually give a lengthy and impressive performance; they sometimes work with a sick person an hour or more at a time.

Barrio people are not in a great hurry about something as sobering as illness. "Efficiency" is not considered a particularly admirable trait. They much prefer that the physician be calm and cautious, and observe the little social proprieties that Mexican-Americans regard as a sign of courtesy and good will. They usually interpret a doctor's haste as rudeness or discourtesy. For a discussion of attitudes toward "efficiency," see the chapter, "Differences in Orientation to Time," in Saunders [43].

Rosenfeld [41] tells the story of a physician in New Mexico who was called out in the middle of the night to see a comatose child. When the doctor arrived at the home of the Spanish-speaking family, the child's mother insisted that they first have a cup of tea. With the unconscious child in the adjoining room, parents and doctor sat in the kitchen and drank their tea. "The conversation was obviously forced—yet . . . one never rushes precipitately into the middle of things; there must be tea and talk before it is proper to examine even a patient as precious as this one. . . . The thoughts of [the mother] were undoubtedly with the sick one, too, as she studied the visitor . . . [she] was not an indifferent mother. But if the doctor was not simpática, how then could she possibly cure the child?" After these preliminaries, the doctor, "trying not to move with a too indecorous haste," was escorted into the next room to examine the unconscious child. The doctor had proved herself a kind and congenial person—the parents knew they could trust her to do the right thing for their child.

All the objections which Mexican-Americans raise to the behavior of physicians apply equally to nurses and other medical personnel. In fact, a nurse may be criticized even more harshly than a physician, perhaps because she more nearly performs the functions of a folk curer, visiting the home and working directly with the patient and his family.

Conflict between lay expectations and the behavior of medical workers is not necessarily confined to Spanish-speaking groups. Although such conflicts may occur in any American community, they are doubly important among immigrant populations who have so many other reasons for rejecting scientific medical care. An English-speaking patient who becomes offended by the authoritarianism, impersonality, or haste of his doctor may merely select another physician. Barrio people, under the same circumstances, often reject doctors altogether and return to the traditional curing ways of their forebears.

8

CHANGING MEDICAL WAYS

THE PRECEDING chapters discussed the social, economic, religious, and folkloric characteristics which affect problems of health and illness in a low-income Mexican-American community. Health workers, for a number of reasons, are seeking a better understanding of these characteristics. Perhaps, through this better understanding, health workers will be able to find a solution to the continuous, serious problems of high incidence of infectious diseases and high morbidity rate among low-income Mexican-Americans. The incidence of some infectious diseases in Spanish-speaking barrios of Santa Clara County, for example, is about four times that of the county as a whole.[1] Such conditions are a health threat to the entire com-

[1] In 1952, 42 per cent of newly reported tuberculosis patients in Santa Clara County were persons of Mexican descent. Since Mexican-Americans constitute only 12 per cent of the total population, the incidence of new cases of this disease was almost four times the normal expectation. (Data supplied by the Division of Statistics, Santa Clara County Public Health Department.)

munity, impair the efficiency of the labor force, raise social-welfare costs, and contribute to human suffering in countless ways.

SUMMARY AND RECOMMENDATIONS

The following discussion summarizes, and recommends ways to overcome, some of the major barriers to better health and longer life for people like Antonio, Marta, and their neighbors.

COMMUNICATION PROBLEMS

Sal si Puedes and other Mayfair barrios are Spanish-speaking communities. Spanish is the primary home language of more than 98 per cent of the population. Spanish is not only the primary language of the people but a symbol of their cultural tradition and of their existence as a social group. About 65 per cent of the people five years of age and older speak some English, but most of these are children and young adults. Even those who can communicate in English are frequently hesitant to speak it and are much more comfortable using their own language. They resent those who criticize them for speaking Spanish (as Antonio resented the nurse who objected to his use of Spanish and told him he must speak English because he was in an American hospital).

A number of adolescents and young adults, however, are sensitive about being ignorant of English. Children and adolescents have a dual language problem arising from an inadequate command of both languages. For this reason they seldom make very good interpreters; they sometimes fail to understand English words or are unable to think of Spanish equivalents. There is usually no way for the monolingual health worker to be sure that proper information has been conveyed by a child translator because the child may try to conceal the fact that he cannot translate adequately.

In Santa Clara County some health workers have used adult bilinguals as translators with good results. One sanitarian has such an arrangement with a Mexican-American grocery clerk in his district who speaks both languages well and also knows most of the neighborhood people. Several child-health conferences have Mexican-American volunteers who can serve as translators.

Barrio people often complain that they cannot get information from hospitals or public health departments by telephone because there is no one available there who understands Spanish. Some complain that switchboard operators cannot understand them and simply break the telephone connection.

A few local hospitals and health departments have Spanish-speaking employees in some capacity (either professional or clerical) who can be called upon when necessary to act as interpreters. At the present time, however, very few medical agencies can provide this service.

A survey of literacy in the community showed that the language barrier extends to the use of written materials. About 75 per cent of the people read some English, but many of these are school children. Only about 50 percent of the adults thirty and older read English. About 16 per cent of the people read Spanish, most of them over thirty-five years of age. About 8 per cent of the people are illiterate and cannot be reached by written materials at all.

Literature may not be understood, even if it can be read, because the wording is too "highbrow" or too technical. Even nontechnical materials may be difficult for the people to read, since those over the age of seventeen have completed an average of only 4.8 years of formal schooling. Technical phrasing may render verbal communication difficult, too. For example, one doctor said to a mother who wanted to wean her child, "Apply a tight pectoral binder and restrict your fluid intake." The woman understood some English, but this scientific jargon was beyond her comprehension. Pride and shyness, however, prevented her asking for an explanation of the doctor's instructions.

The language barrier between medical workers and barrio people shows no sign of being resolved promptly. Even though Spanish-speaking children are now receiving more years of American schooling and are learning more English than did their parents or grandparents, the educational level is rising very slowly. An influx of new Mexican immigrants into the area each year also perpetuates language differences. It is therefore safe to assume that public health workers will continue for some time to face communication problems in dealing with Mexican-American groups.

Recommendations

1. Health workers should "approach" Mexican-Americans cautiously and try to determine which language they prefer to speak. Some may be offended at the suggestion that they do not understand

English. If possible, it is well to use Spanish with patients who obviously prefer that language. Using interpreters is less satisfactory than direct conversation between patient and health worker. Any plan is worthy of consideration which would encourage more public health personnel in Spanish-speaking areas to learn some Spanish.

2. It is recommended that administrators in areas with significant Spanish-speaking groups either consider hiring PBX operators who can receive calls from Spanish-speaking people or make arrangements for relaying such calls to another staff member who can receive messages and supply information in Spanish. These bilingual employees could be called upon when necessary to act as interpreters.

3. It is easy for health workers to overestimate the vocabularies and the scientific knowledge of their clients. Explanations, whether in English or in Spanish, should be simple and free from technical terminology.

4. Reading comprehension in Sal si Puedes is considerably below the level of that of the general public. Health literature aimed at an audience of children or young adults should be in English (preferably not over fourth-grade reading level). Older adults are more likely to read materials in simple Spanish. Materials designed for people of all ages had best be printed in both languages. Common language, however, does not necessarily constitute good communication. Although written materials *should* always be written in terms that the people can understand, they are sometimes not. For example, a pamphlet [11] written in Spanish (in the hope of "communicating" with Mexican-American groups) on the subject of venereal-disease control and circulated in California contains the following expressions: *"infecciones generalizadas"* (generalized infections); *"intervención quirúrgica"* (surgical intervention); *"conformación"* (conformation); *"supuración por la uretra"* (suppuration from the urethra). This medical terminology is unfamiliar to most barrio people and simply has no meaning for them, even though the language used is Spanish.

5. Since language has strong emotional value, it is not advisable to attack language use directly. For example, if hospital patients want to speak Spanish among themselves, they should be allowed to do so. They will feel more at ease and less isolated from their own community. It might be advantageous, in fact, to use bilingual

patients for explaining treatments and procedures to other hospital patients who understand only Spanish.

6. If health programs use mass media, the program planners should consider using not only English channels but also Spanish ones. Radio programs in Spanish are particularly effective in reaching a large audience.

7. If health programs disseminate information through local organizations, some preliminary effort should be made to determine which groups in the community are most influential. These vary from one area to another. In Sal si Puedes, churches and funerarias have greater power to influence behavior than do the more American-type groups (P.T.A., civic organizations) which Anglo health planners usually work with.

8. School children are sometimes used as couriers to carry information back to their parents. Although this procedure is satisfactory for factual reports, it is not very effective for the introduction of new ideas designed to change attitudes or behavior patterns because the young have relatively low status in Mexican-American families. It is recommended that adults be contacted directly whenever possible.

ECONOMIC PROBLEMS

Sal si Puedes people are a low-income group. Those who are eligible for care at the county hospital or in public health clinics usually receive more medical service than those who must go to private physicians. The most acute problems in medical economics are among nonresident seasonal workers and nonindigent families who are struggling to be financially independent. One man reported, "The doctors at the county hospital are good, but it's terrible to try to get past the social workers. You have an awful time getting in, no matter how poor you are. Unless a family is on the county, they can't get in there. One of my friends didn't have a job and no money. The social worker said he couldn't come there but that a private doctor would fix him up for five dollars. He decided he could afford that much so he went to a doctor, but the doctor gave him a bill for twenty-five dollars. These people were really poor and couldn't afford prices like that. One doctor fixed my boy's ear—he saw him just once for about two minutes and gave him a shot—then I got a bill for nine dollars. It's just too expensive to go to a doctor. Poor people can't afford it, but they can't get in the county hospital, either."

Many barrio people reported paying $10 for a single office visit, and $5 was considered a very cheap rate for the San Jose area. People reported paying $15 to $25 for house calls.

The average farm laborer in the area earns between $2,000 and $3,000 annually, with which he must support a family of six to seven. A major illness, a surgical operation, or a period of hospitalization can be an economic disaster. Rather than be faced with medical bills which they cannot pay, many Spanish-speaking families prefer to dispense with a physician's services as long as possible and rely instead on home remedies, folk curers, and marginal practitioners.

Few families have adequate medical insurance, although policies are available to many seasonal workers. For example, the local cannery-workers' union in San Jose has a medical-insurance plan; those who work as much as two or three months a year can retain this coverage by paying the monthly premiums after they stop work. At the present time, most Mexican-American cannery employees fail to take advantage of this opportunity after leaving their jobs at the end of the work season. Several other seasonal industries offer similar medical-insurance plans.

It is important to remember that in the eyes of medical specialists the world revolves around health, but to the patient it is only one of many aspects of everyday life. Time and money are limited for people with low incomes and large families. Money is often the critical factor which determines whether a patient will go to a doctor or do the best he can with the contents of the family medicine chest. If money is desperately needed for other things or if other desires are stronger than the wish to feel a little better, money may be spent for something other than medical care.

Recommendations

1. It is not a simple matter to convince Mexican-Americans of the advantages of pre-payment plans, but there may be some way for public health people to encourage more extensive use of hospitalization plans or health insurance. (For two discussions of some of the problems involved, see Saunders [43] and Saunders and Samora in Paul [37].) Retention of health-plan coverage would prove a great economic advantage to many seasonally employed families.

2. If part-pay clinics or hospitals are available in the area, it is recommended that they be supported and, if possible, their services extended.

3. The problem of transportation to hospitals and clinics is being improved through the establishment of child-health conferences in local communities. An additional possibility might be considered—the extension of medical care to local communities through branch county-hospital clinics in scattered areas. Fresno County, California, has recently established branch county-hospital dispensaries, and initial reports indicate excellent results.

4. Mothers with small children complain of the difficulties they have in keeping medical appointments. Neighborhood coöperative nurseries could perhaps help solve the problem of child care; local service groups might be encouraged to support such projects.

CONFLICTS WITH FOLK BELIEFS

Nonscientific concepts of disease from Mexico are an important influence in the lives of Mexican-Americans. Conflicts between folk beliefs and scientific medical practice can lead to fear and rejection of American health services. Many of these folk beliefs are persistent in second- and third-generation Mexican-Americans. One example is the persistence of beliefs about the importance of dietary restrictions for postpartum mothers. Some women resist hospital deliveries because they are served foods in the hospital which they believe will impair their, or their babies', health in some way.

A second example is the treatment of tuberculosis. There is a widespread belief in Latin America, still held by many Mexican-Americans, that serious illness can be produced by exposure to a current of air; the resulting disease is called mal aire or simply aire (air). Some patients at the county tuberculosis sanatorium, particularly older people, reported that they were terribly afraid of the treatments they were receiving—the aire. It was discovered that the aire referred to was that used in pneumothorax, a treatment which consists of pumping into the patient's chest cavity a quantity of air to restrict the movement of the diseased lung. There are many reasons why Mexican-Americans resist hospitalization for tuberculosis, but one is that some patients consider air to be deadly. If air used in the treatment of tuberculosis were called "oxygen," the danger of confusion with mal aire might be avoided.

Religious beliefs, prayers, and spells of Mexican origin are very important in the diagnosis and home treatment of disease. For example, fragments of holy palm blessed in the church on Palm Sunday are sometimes used to ward off disease or in the magical curing of "evil eye." Another example is the Catholic patient at the county tuberculosis sanatorium who drank a sip of holy water every morning before breakfast.

Among Protestant sects there is emphasis placed on the healing power of God through faith and prayer; some churches have special organizations whose function is helping the sick to be healed through prayer. Some of these sects, representing about 10 per cent of the Mexican-Americans in Mayfair, oppose the use of doctors and hospital facilities on the theory that resorting to medical treatment is an admission of insufficient faith. Most Protestant groups, however, do not discourage the seeking of medical care, maintaining that the doctor is an instrument of God and that God should be allowed to work through His instruments.

Barrio people place considerable reliance on Mexican folk-curing practices such as herbal remedies, "cupping," topical applications of some sort, heat treatments, and massage. Patent medicines are also popular. Barrio people are sometimes afraid of taking strange medicines. One doctor reported that his Mexican-American patients frequently take less than the recommended dose of a prescribed remedy—if the instructions are to take three tablets daily, many patients will take only one or two. An estimated 65 to 70 per cent of all Mexican-American patients who are eventually seen by physicians in San Jose have first tried some other kind of curative measures. One doctor estimated that about 50 per cent of his Spanish-speaking patients have first consulted some other type of curer—herbalist, curandera, chiropractor, or homeopath. One patient who was discovered to have advanced tuberculosis had been under the care of a Chinese herbalist for three years. The popularity of marginal practitioners is due in part to their use of curative procedures which are not unfamiliar to Mexican folk medicine.

It should be emphasized that folk syndromes are very real to barrio people. Health workers who flatly deny the existence of "evil eye," mal aire, empacho, "magical fright," or disease caused by witchcraft may expect to lose the confidence of many of their Mexican-American patients. Perhaps a greater tolerance and understanding of folk beliefs may be fostered if health workers recall that modern medical practice also has its remnants of folklore and that, as Parsons [36] points out, "the institutionalization of science is . . .

far from complete within the profession . . . as evidenced by the strong, often bitter resistance from within the profession itself to the acceptance of what have turned out to be critically important scientific advances in their own field."

Recommendations

1. It is recommended that medical workers try to learn something about local medical beliefs and practices in order to gain stature, to avoid appearing ignorant, and to be enabled to work toward dispelling those folk customs which are detrimental. The use of ridicule should be avoided in all situations. With those who are convinced of the validity of their beliefs it might be possible to work within the context of folk medicine. For example, if a mother suggests that her child is suffering from "fallen fontanelle," a doctor or nurse might point out that Anglos call this disorder by another name—dehydration. Differences in ideas of etiology might simply be ignored. Conflict might also be avoided by saying, "Yes, I know about that disease, but it seems to me that this is something else." Foster [17] has made the following suggestion:

If an obviously sick child suffering from fever, headache, and vomiting were brought to the doctor, and the mother did not hesitate to say "I suspect it is the evil eye," the doctor should lose none of his professional integrity by replying, "Well, let's see. There are many illnesses with similar symptoms, and my examination convinces me that in this case it is such and such, and I recommend the following treatment." The doctor is neither ridiculing nor sanctioning the mother's belief—he is diplomatically bypassing it. As a specialist he points out why it is more likely to be something else, and as a sympathetic specialist his advice may very well be followed.

2. Since there is strong faith in the healing powers of herbal remedies it might be advisable, in encouraging the use of prescribed medication, to explain that drugs are often made from herbs: "Doctors have found that such and such an herb was an excellent remedy for this condition; the medicine I am giving you is made from that herb, but it is much purer than the crude plant." The suggestion has been made that if a child is to be given large quantities of boiled water in the treatment of diarrhea, it is advisable to prescribe instead large volumes of herbal teas. Mothers may not see the value in forcing plain water on the infant, but they have confidence in the

value of herbal teas and will be much more likely to follow the instructions [17].

3. Medical workers should recognize the strength of religious convictions among many of their Mexican-American patients, particularly those who rely on faith healing. There seems to be no need for health workers to secularize everything. Sneering at faith healing can drive away devoutly religious patients who might gladly come to be cured if the physician were willing to let them regard him as an instrument of God.

4. Health workers dealing with problems of nutritional deficiency should not try to encourage sudden and marked changes in diet. Better results can be obtained by recommending the use of different proportions of foods already in the local diet.

5. It is recommended that simple Mexican foods be served in hospitals to Mexican-American patients more frequently—for example, Spanish rice, pinto beans, tortillas, and hot chili sauce. If chili sauce could be provided to Mexican-American patients regularly as a condiment (as catsup is served to Anglo), many foods otherwise thought tasteless could be enjoyed.

6. Mexican-American postpartum mothers complain that they are served foods in the hospital which are "bad" for them because they are "too hot" or "too cold" (see table 8). It might be well to avoid serving these foods (e.g., pork, tomato juice) too frequently or, at least, to provide a choice of dietary items so that Mexican-American women would not be forced either to go hungry or to violate food taboos.

PROBLEMS RELATED TO DEFINITIONS OF DISEASE

Spanish-speaking people and Anglo medical personnel sometimes have different conceptions of normal and abnormal physical states. There are, for example, differences in what is considered "normal" growth and development. Marta, for example, was indignant when a district nurse told her that her baby was not able to walk soon enough because he was too fat. From Marta's point of view the child was not too fat but normal and healthy. She deeply resented the suggestion that her baby was abnormal or retarded in his motor development.

In Sal si Puedes illness is generally defined as a state of bodily discomfort. A person who has no debilitating symptoms is usually held to be well and healthy even though the diagnostic tests of scientific practitioners may reveal such serious pathological processes as carcinoma, tuberculosis, or heart disease. It is difficult for the people to understand how a sick person can feel well and go about his normal tasks without discomfort. To say to a patient without symptoms, "You are sick," is to invite confusion and disbelief.

The "preclinical" stage of illness is a concept which is familiar in folk belief; for example, a person may not develop the symptoms of susto for some time after the frightening episode which produces the illness. If prophylactic measures are taken during this time, the disease may be avoided. It is not clear just why the preclinical stages of scientific syndromes are not recognized. Perhaps it is simply because the situation has not been presented to the people in familiar terms.

Since the community defines disease as the presence of symptoms, there is sometimes grave concern over the significance of unusual bodily states which medical specialists view as "functional variations within the normal range." A Spanish-speaking patient may consult a physician for symptoms such as insomnia, anxiety, or "nervousness." A child with "sad eyes" or one who "doesn't sleep enough" may be taken for medical treatment whereas one with diarrhea, a common condition in the barrio, may not be considered particularly ill. A thin man whose lack of abdominal fat permits the palpation of the abdominal aorta may promptly seek treatment for latido, a dread folk disease; but a person who has night sweats and a persistent cough is likely to be treated with home remedies for "a little cold." Coughing and sweating are everyday occurrences in the barrio, but a "pounding stomach" is a strange and frightening phenomenon.

Physicians are sometimes annoyed with the naïveté of Mexican-American patients about what medical science regards as "significant" symptoms. It may be of some consolation to the harassed health worker to remember that he makes a real contribution by assuring his patients that their complaints, while disconcerting, have no ominous meaning.

Recommendations

1. The preclinical stage of illness should be carefully explained. A good approach might be to inform asymptomatic patients (for

example, those with minimal tuberculosis) that of course they feel well now but that they have been exposed to a dangerous illness which is attacking their bodies and that unless they receive prompt treatment they will become very sick indeed.

2. From the patient's point of view, reassurance that his symptoms are not pathological may be as important as the diagnosis and treatment of "real" disease.

One of the most frequent complaints that Mexican-American patients make about medical treatment is that it is embarrassing. Girls and women, particularly, are extremely modest—it is a pattern taught them from childhood. One young woman reported that she had never undressed in the presence of her sisters. She would not think of removing even her outer garments unless she were alone. This is a general attitude which makes it difficult for Spanish-speaking patients to expose their bodies even to medical workers.

A young mother in east San Jose took her infant son to a child-health conference. The child was discovered to have a stricture of the foreskin which interferred with complete emptying of the bladder. The public health physician asked the mother, in a rather abrupt manner, "Why haven't you had this child circumcised?" The woman, surprised and embarrassed by the question, was unable to answer the doctor. The question was repeated and the mother became somewhat defensive. Finally the clinic nurse interposed with the suggestion that if the mother did not want the child to have surgery she might help the condition by manual manipulation which little by little would ease the stricture. The mother, horrified by the suggestion, asserted, "I'm not going to touch it!"

This conflict might have been avoided had the health workers been aware of the extreme modesty of most Mexican-American women. Asking a mother to handle the genitalia of her male infant except when cleanliness demands it is asking that she perform what she considers an indecent act. The child's father, however, could have been asked to perform the manipulation without such moral indignation.

Doctors and nurses in the fields of obstetrics, gynecology, and venereal-disease control are made acutely aware of the problems stemming from the Mexican-American concept of modesty. It is in these fields that modesty problems most often arise, and special care must be taken to avoid serious damage to medical relationships.

Recommendations

1. Health workers should try to avoid embarrassing patients: for example, more bodily exposure than absolutely necessary should be avoided; beds in hospitals should be screened during any period of body exposure; sexual topics should not be discussed in mixed groups; in venereal-disease control, private conferences are advisable.

2. Because Mexican-American women and girls are extremely modest, it is advisable to consult with fathers, rather than mothers, concerning genitourinary problems of male children.

PROBLEMS RELATED TO MEDICAL ROLES

Different cultures have different conceptions of the proper roles played by participants in medical situations. For example, many Anglos who have become increasingly aware of preventive medicine and hygiene accept the idea that some disease is the result of neglect or carelessness on the part of the patient or those responsible for his welfare. Mexican-Americans, on the other hand, rarely blame patients for getting sick, nor do patients feel guilty or responsible for an illness. A medical worker who implies that a sick person is at fault and is somehow responsible for his condition may find his statements received with indignation or hostility. To the patient and his family, such a view is unjust or even malicious.

The Anglo medical practitioner is taught that an impersonal objectivity is a vital part of his role as an applied scientist. He places a premium on "efficiency"—he tries to "come directly to the point," dispense with "unnecessary" formalities, and achieve maximum output in minimum time. He assumes also that his status as a trained specialist gives prestige and authority to his opinions and his recommendations.

The people of Sali si Puedes, however, expect quite different behavior from therapists. Their expectations are based largely on the usual behavior patterns of Mexican folk curers. People who expect a curer to be warm, friendly, and interested in all aspects of the patient's life find it difficult to trust a doctor who is impersonal and "clinical" in his manner. Nor do they accept his authority to "give

orders." He may suggest or counsel, but an authoritarian or dictatorial approach on his part is resented and rejected. His behavior,
culturally sanctioned in his own society, is often interpreted by
Spanish-speaking patients as discourtesy if not outright boorishness.

Family members take a much more active role in medical care
than they do in most Anglo communities. Two full days' observation
in the waiting room of the Santa Clara County Hospital Clinic, for
example, *disclosed not a single Mexican-American patient unaccom-
panied by friends or relatives.* In one private physician's office an
elderly male patient was accompanied by two sons, a daughter-in-
law, and a grandson. In Mexican-American families the patient alone
does not make medical decisions; his relatives and compadres may
be the ones to decided on a course of action. Relatives expect to
retain control over the treatment of disease and resent relinquishing
this control to strangers who have no personal interest in the patient's welfare. Patients, too, resent having their families excluded
from medical situations; they often resist hospitalization because it
means isolation from the attentions and moral support of their
kinsmen and compadres.

Recommendations

1. It is not advisable to expect a patient to make a medical decision until he has had a chance to consult with family members.
Medical workers should avoid approaches which fix individual responsibility; group responsibility should be recognized. It is desirable
for public health workers to make an effort to consult with those
of the patient's family who have real authority in the group. For
example, if possible, a child's health problems should be discussed
with both parents. The mother alone may not have authority to act
in the child's behalf. If a patient is accompanied to a clinic or a
doctor's office by other family members, it is well to inquire about
their relationship to the patient and to consult with them about the
patient's welfare. District nurses are wise to determine some of the
compadrazgo relationships of their clients; if there is difficulty in
getting coöperation from the patient or his immediate family, compadres may be willing to use their influence in getting the patient
to take medical action. It is advisable to try to include an older
person in a family discussion. A grandmother, for example, can be
a powerful influence in medical decisions.

It may be best to encourage whole families or groups of families to adopt a new health program, rather than putting pressure on a single individual, who may be more afraid of what people will say than of what the doctor may think. In most public health services there are time, space, and personnel limitations which make it hard for doctors or nurses to work with whole groups of people at one time. Public health projects, however, can be much more effective if an approach is used which includes whole family groups.

2. It is well to remember that people have problems other than medical ones, and that their responsibilities to family or other social groups may supersede medical demands. Sometimes the effort of a public health worker to help a client get a boy out of juvenile hall or locate a job, for example, may clear the way for tackling medical problems.

3. A cold and impersonal approach to Mexican-American clients should by all means be avoided. A barrio patient does not trust medical workers who are unfriendly, but has confidence in those who seem sincerely interested in him, in his family, and in his feelings. If patients seem ill at ease or disturbed, it might be well to ask frankly, "Are you afraid of something? What can I do to help you to feel better about this?"

4. A patient or his family should not be scolded or blamed for an illness. If it is thought that the disorder is due to real negligence, it is advisable to wait until the illness is under control and then say, "We have learned that there is a way to prevent this happening again. Would you like me to tell you about it so that you can protect your family?" It is advisable to stress the positive advantages to be gained from following a proposed course of action rather than antagonizing the client by pointing to his failures or omissions.

PROBLEMS OF SOCIAL DISTANCE

Health specialists who work with Spanish-speaking communities are set apart socially from their clients. Three factors of the public health worker's status maintain social distance between him and the people with whom he deals: First, he is a government employee and as such is related to other government workers—law-enforcement officers, tax assessors, immigration authorities, truant officers, building inspectors, FBI agents, and public prosecutors—all of whom are viewed as potential threats to the security of barrio people.

Although the Santa Clara County Public Health Department has made an effort to separate itself in the minds of the people from law-enforcement agencies, there is still some fear in the community that public health workers may be secretly in league with other government agents who could "cause trouble." One woman, for example, was frightened by the prospect of a home visit from the district nurse: "You know we've got a lot of relatives staying with us now, and if that nurse finds out that we've got fifteen people living here in three rooms, she'll surely go to the welfare office—then they'll call our landlord and have us put out in the street." This fearful prediction did not materialize, of course, but it does illustrate the uneasy feeling that public health workers are outsiders and are not to be trusted.

The second factor which maintains the gulf between medical workers and Spanish-speaking clients is that most public health people are Anglos. Aside from the communication barriers that result from this difference, there are also conflicts resulting from historic group tensions between Anglos and Mexican-Americans in California and parts of the Southwest. Barrio people are members of a minority group in the United States. Many of them have lived in localities (as the Texas-Mexico border area or the urban Los Angeles vicinity) where, in the past, group tensions have been acute and have sometimes involved open violence. For this reason many Mexican-Americans feel hostile toward Anglos. Those who are not actually hostile may at least feel uncomfortable with English-speaking persons, fear discriminatory treatment, and remain acutely sensitive to Anglo criticism.

It has been suggested that Mexican-American communities should be served by Spanish-speaking public health workers. There is much merit in this recommendation; many medical specialists of Mexican descent in California are working effectively and making significant contributions in public health fields. The use of Spanish-speaking personnel offers a ready solution to many problems of communication and interethnic conflict.

It should be mentioned, however, that the employment of Mexican-American personnel is not a complete solution to the problem of social distance. The third factor, that of socioeconomic class difference, is also to be considered.

The class differences which characterize the Spanish-speaking colony in San Jose have been discussed in chapter 2. Mexican-American doctors, nurses, and medical social workers are professionals and thus, by definition, members of la alta sociedad, or "high society," in the colony. Residents of Sal si Puedes, on the other hand, consider themselves los medianos, a lower social grade. There is a great deal of resentment in the barrio toward some "successful" Mexican-Americans who are thought to turn traitor to their own people and identify themselves with the Anglo community.

Some Mexican-American professionals have successfully bridged the class barrier and have achieved acceptance in low-income neighborhoods. But unless Spanish-speaking medical workers are extremely careful to avoid a supercilious, an overbearing, or a patronizing attitude, they may achieve less rapport with barrio people than do those Anglos who are able to overcome language and ethnic differences with friendliness, courtesy, and an honest respect for the dignity of their Spanish-speaking neighbors.

Recommendations

1. It is well to avoid offending group loyalties by using approaches which conspicuously indicate that Mexican-Americans are basically different in some way from other people. Such approaches may be interpreted as discriminatory. Spatial segregation in hospitals and clinics should be discouraged, for example. As indicated previously, it is often necessary to cater to special Mexican-American problems; however, workers should try to do this inconspicuously so that it will not occur to the patient that he is receiving unusual treatment but merely that he is dealing with friendly helpful people.

2. Program planners will find it advantageous to discover the persons of prestige or power in the local community and enlist their support in public health programs (priests, ministers, neighborhood "leaders"). It should be remembered that those whom Anglos regard as "Mexican leaders" may be thought of as "big shots" or "outsiders" to members of the target group. Such people may not be well accepted among their own people. A health program can prove ineffective simply because barrio people resent having their affairs turned over to outsiders. Those who are effective leaders in their own neighborhoods may be harder to find and more difficult for Anglos to work with; efforts to gain their coöperation and support, however, are rarely wasted.

3. Medical personnel can often minimize their social distance from patients by avoiding patronizing attitudes or authoritarian approaches. Health workers need not hesitate to make friends with patients and to take a personal interest in their affairs. A little extra time taken for social amenities is well spent. District workers, for example, should accept food or drink if it is offered. They should not enter a home, however, until they are specifically invited. This time investment in the initial stages of a medical relationship may actually save time later. A public health worker who shows courtesy and graciousness will be accepted as a warm and congenial person who can be trusted and whose suggestions must be considered. District nurses might consider the possibility of attending local gatherings occasionally in order to show their sincere interest in the community and its people. Even clinic physicians and nurses may be able to establish friendly relations by taking a little time at the beginning of an interview to socialize with patients.

THE PROBLEM OF HOSPITALIZATION

Some of the reasons barrio people generally dread and fear hospitalization are: lack of understanding of the reasons for treatment or other hospital procedures, isolation from family and friends, fear of the unknown, fear of inability to communicate their needs to hospital workers, fear of discriminatory treatment, fear of affronts to modesty or individual dignity, unaccustomed diet, and inability to meet family responsibilities while in the hospital. All of these have been discussed earlier as reasons for resistance to public health programs. For many Spanish-speaking patients, hospitalization represents the synthesis of all the most objectionable aspects of Anglo medical care.

Recommendations

1. Until some of these problems are resolved, it is advisable to allow Mexican-American patients to be cared for at home whenever possible.

2. If hospital admission cannot be avoided because of the severity or infectious nature of the illness, patients should be allowed to have relatives with them as often as possible and should be placed where they may converse with other Spanish-speaking patients. Com-

plete segregation, however, should be discouraged for reasons discussed above.

CONCLUSION

Changes in medical beliefs and practices are coming about in the barrios of the Mayfair community. Scientific medical practice is making slow inroads into the thinking and customs of the people.

There are still many Mexican folk remedies used in San Jose, but a change is taking place in the minds of the people about their use. For example, dietary restrictions and herbal remedies are still in vogue, but many people have forgotten (or never learned) the folk theories underlying their use. A person born and reared in Mexico can usually explain why it is bad for a postpartum mother to eat pork—it is a "very hot" food. A second-generation Mexican-American may cling to the belief that pork is "bad" for new mothers, but frequently cannot explain why. A third-generation American is likely to say something like this: "People say that pork isn't good for a new mother, but when my baby was born I ate some and it didn't make me sick."

The theory of "hot and cold," one of the most dominant medical beliefs in Latin America, is gradually being reinterpreted in Mexican-American communities. Although the people often talk about the "heat" and "cold" of foods, medicines, or bodily states, they are coming to think more in terms of actual temperatures rather than "qualities" or "essences." This modification of folk belief renders ideas about illness and its treatment more compatible with scientific theory and practice (for example, our treatment of fever by cold compresses or cold alcohol rubs).

There is a general "loss" of the theory underlying herbal lore. Although some of the older women of the barrios have retained a considerable knowledge of herbs, most people use herbal remedies rather indiscriminately without a real understanding of why they are used. In the absence of Mexican yerbalistas in San Jose, there is a tendency to patronize Chinese herb doctors.

There is the same lack of understanding in the use of new medicines. For example, Lupe explained that Anglo doctors had given her sister a red medicine to drink as a treatment for goiter. It was the same medicine, she said, "that you use on cuts and that the doctors put on your skin when you have an operation." She obviously was referring to merthiolate, which was certainly not the medication her sister received orally (the medication actually prescribed was elixir of phenobarbital). Lupe had accepted merthiolate as a "good medicine" without having the vaguest idea of its pharmaceutical properties or the limits of its utility.

A general practitioner in San Jose reported that some of his patients expect to be given either a prescription or a hypodermic injection during an office visit. Even though a patient's condition might not require an injection, he has accepted the idea that "shots are good"; if the doctor fails to administer this beneficial treatment, he has not "done everything possible" for the patient. He leaves the doctor's office feeling that he has somehow been cheated or that his condition has been neglected. This view of shots is not a universal pattern in the barrio, but is common enough to warrant comment.

Empirical evidence seems to be primarily responsible for the acceptance of medical changes in Sal si Puedes. Foster [17] has said that "the average Latin American is pragmatic by nature," and that scientific medical care can best be "sold" to people by repeated demonstrations that doctors know what they are doing and can and do cure disease. The same pragmatism prevails among Mexican-Americans in Sal si Puedes; if they are shown frequently and dramatically that certain procedures effect cures, they eventually become convinced. Elvira, for example, came to reject the Mexican folk belief that if a pregnant woman ate chilies, her baby would have chincual, or diaper rash; her conclusion was based on empirical evidence—"I always ate hot chilies, and none of my babies ever had it." The willingness of people to change their beliefs and practices in the light of convincing evidence has led to the acceptance of many methods of scientific medical practice—immunizations against various childhood diseases, antibiotics for pneumonia and other acute infections, insulin for diabetes, and surgery for appendicitis.

Many people, however, remain skeptical about the wisdom of making extensive use of the physician's services. Barrio people tell many stories about sick people who failed to recover in spite of medical care. They are impressed with the number of diseases for which scientific medicine still has no cure. In some cases even successful treatment may not impress the patient or his family because many patients simultaneously receive folk medication, and the latter is given credit for the cure. It may be that a patient failed to improve even with a physician's care because treatment was abandoned prematurely; if no immediate results were seen, the treatment was therefore assumed to be ineffectual. There are, of course, no rapid and dramatic recoveries from such disorders as tuberculosis or heart disease. For chronic illness, therefore, there is generally less acceptance of the value of scientific treatment simply because the patient's improvement is so gradual and unimpressive.

Acceptance of scientific medicine in Mayfair is increasing slowly and is far from complete. The transition from the use of folk medicine to the acceptance of scientific medical care is retarded by the constant influx of new immigrants entering the community from Mexico or from migratory life which affords few opportunities for learning American ways. There are families who become almost fully assimilated into Anglo culture, but these people generally move away from the barrios and into predominantly Anglo areas. The homes which they vacate are often filled by new Mexican immigrants or by previously migratory families who bring with them a strong Mexican folk tradition. The constant shifting in the composition of the group makes assimilation more difficult.

Other factors oppose acceptance of Anglo medical patterns. Some of these are: the insularity of the community with its partial spatial segregation, language difference, and fear of discrimination or insult by Anglos; strong loyalties to the family and the neighborhood group and the desire to avoid conflict with group members; a fear of shame or ridicule for departure from cultural traditions; the dream of many older folk of someday returning to Mexico (which encourages the persistence of values oriented toward Mexican goals); and fear and suspicion of the unknown and untried.

On the other hand, there are features of American life that barrio people like and want for themselves, features which serve to motivate people toward change to Anglo patterns. For example, they want a higher standard of living—better jobs, better homes, more money; they want the higher social status which comes to those who learn and practice Anglo ways; they want many of the "created needs" fostered by American advertising—cars, television sets, refrigerators, and encyclopedias.

Public health programs aimed at Spanish-speaking groups must utilize the positive motivations toward change and avoid the negative ones. On the basis of the social and cultural information gathered for this book, it has been possible to suggest ways in which public health workers can deal more effectively with Mexican-American communities, like the barrios of Mayfair, and thus speed the acceptance and use of American health facilities.

ahijado, ahijada—godson, goddaughter.

alta sociedad—"high society"; upper class.

angelito—little angel; children who have not yet been confirmed in the Catholic religion. They are thought to go at death directly to Heaven rather than having to pass through purgatory.

angina(s)—sore throat; tonsillitis.

asustado—"frightened" (see *susto*).

atole—thin gruel of corn meal or other cereal prepared with water or milk; chocolate or other flavoring is sometimes added.

baile—ball or public dance.

baile de quince—debut; a formal ball and party at which a girl who has reached her fifteenth birthday is presented to society; the custom is almost defunct in San Jose.

barrio—neighborhood; ward. The term is usually applied only to areas which are largely Spanish-speaking.

bilis—"bile"; a folk-disease thought to result from unusual anger or rage.

bolito—little ball.

bolo—a child's ball; also, figuratively, small gifts or coins given to children of a parish by a godfather after Catholic baptism.

braceros—Mexican nationals brought into the United States as contract farm laborers during the harvest season.

bruja—female witch.

brujería—witchcraft.

Calvario—Calvary; a raised mound of earth on which is placed the Cross during the *Vía Crucis* (*q.v.*).

campesinos—rustics; countryfolk.

Candelaria—Candlemas.

cantina—saloon, barroom.

cargueros—men responsible for the care of images of the saints in Mexican village churches.

catarro constipado—head cold.

charros—Mexican riders known for feats of horsemanship and their typical costume, elaborate cowboy clothing.

chicano—a Mexican-American (slang).

chiles bravos—extremely hot peppers.

China Poblana—type of female Mexican folk costume characterized by

241

white peasant blouse and full skirt highly embroidered with satin threads or sequins. This costume is associated with the Mexican image of the ideal woman.

chincual—disease of infants, characterized by redness and pustules on the buttocks; diaper rash. Thought to be caused by the mother's eating "hot" foods during pregnancy.

Cinco de Mayo—Fifth of May; Mexican Independence Day.

colonia—colony; specifically, the Mexican-American community within a particular urban area.

comadre—"comother"; the godmother of one's child or the mother of one's godchild.

compadrazgo—the system of formalized friendships or artificial kin relationships between parents and godparents and brought into play through various Catholic sacraments.

compadre—"cofather"; the godfather of one's child or the father of one's godchild.

con nalgas adelante—breech presentation in childbirth.

Cristo—Christ.

cuarentena—period of forty days following childbirth. During this time a woman, ideally, is expected to remain in partial confinement and carefully restrict her diet and activities.

Cuaresma—Lent.

cumpleaños—birthday.

curandera—curing woman; Mexican folk curer.

descalzo—barefoot.

Día de los Santos Reyes—Day of the Holy Kings (January 6); Epiphany, the end of the Catholic Christmas season.

Día de Todos Santos—Feast of All Saints (November 1).

empacho—"surfeit"; in Mexican folk belief, a stomach disorder caused by eating too much of certain foods. It is characterized by the formation of a hard "ball" inside the stomach.

enfriamiento—"cold" in a joint or other body part.

fiestas patrias—Mexican national holidays, May 5 and September 16.

funeraria—burial society.

gabacho(a)—derogatory slang expression for an Anglo-American.

gringo—Anglo-American.

indio—Indian.

jamaica—church bazaar or "social" at which food is sold and games, dances, music, and other festivities are held.

latido—"palpitation"; a dreaded folk disease characterized by loss of appetite and a "pounding stomach."

los de abajo—the lowly ones; lower class.

Los de Don—those with the gift; a special group within a San Jose Pentecostal sect who pray for the sick and are thought especially gifted in faith healing.

madrina—godmother.

mal aire—"bad air"; a folk disease attributed to sudden exposure to drafts or winds.

mal ojo—"evil eye"; a folk disease attributed to magical causes and to which children are thought particularly susceptible.

mañanitas—a special Catholic mass in honor of the Virgin.

manda—religious vow or promise.

medianos—the middle ones; middle class.

menudo—Mexican tripe soup.

Misa de Gloria—Easter Mass.

mollera caída—"fallen fontanelle"; in folk belief, a disease of infants caused by the "dropping" of the part of the head directly underneath the anterior fontanelle.

mono—dummy; effigy.

nervio—nerve; sometimes, the germinal tissue of an egg.

nopalitos—diced prickly-pear cactus; a popular vegetable dish.

novena—the nine nights following a funeral mass: on each night a rosary is said in honor of the deceased.

pachuco—Mexican-American adolescent characterized by dress and speech (a special argot); in popular Anglo-American thought a term synonymous with Spanish-speaking juvenile delinquent.

padrastrito—little stepfather; a term sometimes used in reference to an older brother.

padre—father; a priest.

padrino—godfather.

pan dulce—Mexican sweet yeast roll.

partera—midwife.

pastorela—Christmas pageant.

Pastores, Los—The Shepherds; a *pastorela* (*q.v.*).

patrón—landlord; patron; employer.

piñata—highly decorated container (usually a clay jar) filled with candy and toys at Christmas; the breaking of the *piñata* is a Christmas game for children.

pocho—an American-born person of Mexican descent (slang).

Posadas, Las—"inns" or "lodgings"; a pre-Christmas ceremonial.

Protestantes—Protestants.

remedios—remedies; medicines.

resfriado—head cold.

ruleta—roulette or "wheel of fortune"; a popular game at *jamaicas* (*q.v.*).

Sábado de Gloria—Easter Saturday.

Sal si Puedes—"Get out if you can"; popular name of a San Jose *barrio* (*q.v.*).

San Antonio—Saint Anthony, patron of domestic animals; also, name of a San Jose *barrio* (*q.v.*).

San Blas—Saint Blaise, patron of throats.

santo—saint; the image of a saint.

Santo Niño de Atocha—Holy Child of Atocha; Spanish saint credited with many miraculous cures.

sobada—massage.

Sociedad Guadalupana—Guadalupe Society, a Catholic women's organization.

susto—"fright"; a folk disease attributed to sudden or prolonged terror.

tecolote—owl; in Mexico, a bird of ill omen.

tonto—an ignorant person; a "country hick."

tortilla—a thin round cake of either corn meal or wheat flour; the typical form of bread made in Mexico.

tortillería—tortilla factory.

tradiciones—traditions; customs.

velorio—a wake.

ventosas—"cupping"; a form of medical therapy.

Vía Crucis—"Way of the Cross," a Catholic Good Friday procession.

viejitos—elderly people.

Virgen de Guadalupe—Virgin of Guadalupe, patroness of Mexico.

BIBLIOGRAPHY

[1] Barker, George C. "Social Functions of Language in a Mexican-American Community," *Acta Americana*, 5 (1947): 185–202.

[2] ———. *Pachuco: An American-Spanish Argot and its Social Function in Tucson, Arizona.* Tucson, University of Arizona Social Science Bulletin 18, 1950.

[3] Beals, Ralph. *Cheran: A Sierra Tarascan Village.* Washington, D. C., Publications of the Institute of Social Anthropology, Smithsonian Institution, no. 2, 1946.

[4] ———. "Culture Patterns of Mexican-American Life," *Proceedings of the Fifth Annual Conference, Southwestern Conference on the Education of Spanish-Speaking People* (Los Angeles, January, 1951), pp. 5–13.

[5] Bogardus, Emory S. "Gangs of Mexican-American Youth," *Sociology and Social Research*, 28 (1943): 55–66.

[6] Brand, Donald D. *Quiroga, A Mexican Municipio.* Washington, D. C., Publications of the Institute of Social Anthropology, Smithsonian Institution, no. 11, 1951.

[7] Broom, Leonard, and Eshref Shevky. "Mexicans in the United States: A Problem in Social Differentiation," *Sociology and Social Research*, 36 (1952): 150–158.

[8] Burma, John M. *Spanish Speaking Groups in the United States.* Durham, Duke University Press, 1954.

[9] California State Department of Finance. Estimate released December 2, 1955 (*Oakland Tribune*, December 2, 1955).

[10] California State Department of Public Health, Nutrition Service. *Highlights, Dietary Survey, 1955: Mayfair Elementary School, Santa Clara County, California*, p. 9 (mimeographed).

[11] California State Department of Public Health, Venereal Disease Service, San Francisco. *Tiene Usted Dos Enemigos!*

[12] Campa, Arthur L. "Some Herbs and Plants of Early California," *Western Folklore*, 9 (1950): 338–347.

246 Bibliography

[13] Curtin, L. S. M. *Healing Herbs of the Rio Grande.* Sante Fe, Laboratory of Anthropology, 1947.

[14] De Treviño, Elizabeth B. "My Heart Lies South," *Woman's Home Companion* (August, 1953), 32 ff.

[15] Devereaux, George, and F. R. Weiner. "The Occupational Status of Nurses," *American Sociological Review,* 15 (1950): 628–634.

[16] Foster, George M. *Empire's Children: The People of Tzintzuntzan.* Washington, D. C., Publications of the Institute of Social Anthropology, Smithsonian Institution, no. 6, 1948.

[17] ———. "Relationships Between Theoretical and Applied Anthropology: A Public Health Program Analysis," *Human Organization,* 11 (1952): 5–16.

[18] ———. "Relationships Between Spanish and Spanish-American Folk Medicine," *Journal of American Folklore,* 66 (1953): 201–217.

[19] ———. "Working with People of Different Cultural Backgrounds," *California's Health,* 13 (1956): 107–110.

[20] Foster, George M., and John H. Rowe. "Suggestions for Field Recording of Information on the Hippocratic Classification of Diseases and Remedies," *Kroeber Anthropological Society Papers,* no. 5 (1951): 1–5.

[21] Fuller, Varden, John W. Mainer, and George L. Viles. *Domestic and Imported Workers in the Harvest Labor Market, Santa Clara County, California, 1954.* University of California, Giannini Foundation of Agricultural Economics, Report no. 184, 1956 (mimeographed).

[22] Gamio, Manuel. *The Mexican Immigrant—His Life Story.* Chicago, University of Chicago Press, 1931.

[23] Gillin, John. "Magical Fright," *Psychiatry,* 11 (1948): 387–400.

[24] Hall, Frederic. *The History of San Jose and Surroundings.* San Francisco, A. L. Bancroft and Co., 1871.

[25] Harvey, Louise F. "The Delinquent Mexican Boy," *Journal of Educational Research,* 42 (1949): 573–585.

[26] Henderson, L. J. "The Patient and Physician as a Social System," *New England Journal of Medicine,* 212 (1935): 819–823.

[27] Humphrey, Normal D. "Some Dietary and Health Practices of Detroit Mexicans," *Journal of American Folklore,* 58 (1945): 255–258.

[28] ———. "The Cultural Background of the Mexican Immigrant," *Rural Sociology,* 13 (1948): 239–255.

[29] Kelly, Isabel. *An Anthropological Approach to Midwifery Training.* Institute of Inter-American Affairs, Mexico, D. F., 1954 (mimeographed).

[30] Lee, A. M. "The Social Dynamics of the Physician's Status," *Psychiatry,* 7 (1944): 371–377.

[31] McDonogh, Edward C. "Status Levels of Mexicans," *Sociology and Social Research,* 33 (1949): 449–459.

[32] Madsen, William. "Hot and Cold in the Universe of San Francisco Tecospa, Valley of Mexico," *Journal of American Folklore,* 68 (1955): 123–139.

[33] Murray, Sister Mary John. *A Socio-Cultural Study of 118 Mexican Families Living in a Low-rent Public Housing Project in San Antonio, Texas.* Washington, D. C., Catholic University of America Press, 1954.

[34] Parsons, Elsie C. *Mitla, Town of the Souls.* Chicago, University of Chicago Press, 1936.

[35] Parsons, Talcott. "Illness and the Role of the Physician: A Sociological Perspective," *American Journal of Orthopsychiatry,* 21 (1951): 452–460.

[36] ———. *The Social System.* London, Tavistock Publications, Ltd., 1952.

[37] Paul, Benjamin D. (ed.). *Health, Culture and Community; Case Studies of Public Reactions to Health Programs.* New York, Russell Sage Foundation, 1955.

[38] Redfield, Robert. *Tepoztlan: A Mexican Village.* Chicago, University of Chicago Press, 1930.

[39] ———. *The Folk Culture of Yucatan.* Chicago, University of Chicago Press, 1941.

[40] Redfield, Robert, and Margaret P. Redfield. *Disease and its Treatment in Dzitas, Yucatan.* Washington, D. C., Carnegie Institution of Washington Publications, vol. 6, no. 32 (Contributions to American Anthropology and History, no. 523), 1940.

[41] Rosenfeld, Albert. "Modern Medicine Where 'The Clock Walks,'" *Collier's Magazine* (February 3, 1956), 24–29.

[42] Santa Clara County Office of Vital Statistics, San Jose, California, April, 1955. Personal communication.

[43] Saunders, Lyle. *Cultural Differences and Medical Care: The Case of the Spanish-speaking People of the Southwest.* New York, Russell Sage Foundation, 1954.

[44] Simmons, Ozzie G. "Popular and Modern Medicine in Mestizo Communities of Coastal Peru and Chile," *Journal of American Folklore,* 65 (1955): 57–71.

[45] Stone, Adolf (ed.). *California Almanac and State Fact Book: 1953–1954.* California Almanac Co., Maywood, California.

[46] Thompson and West. *Historical Atlas Map of Santa Clara County, California.* San Francisco (privately printed), 1876.

[47] Toor, Frances. *A Treasury of Mexican Folkways.* New York, Crown Publishers, 1947.

[48] Tuck, Ruth D. *Not with the Fist: Mexican-Americans in a Southwest City.* New York, Harcourt, Brace and Co., 1946.

[49] U. S. Bureau of the Census. *Census of Population: 1950.* Census Tract Statistics: San Jose, California, vol. 3, chap. 50, "Table 6.—Characteristics of the White Population with Spanish Surname, for Selected Tracts: 1950," p. 22. Washington, D. C., U. S. Government Printing Office, 1952.

[50] U. S. Bureau of the Census. *Census of Population: 1950.* Special Reports, vol. 4, part 3, chap. C, Persons of Spanish Surname, p. 43. Washington, D. C., U. S. Government Printing Office, 1953.

[51] Van der Eerden, M. Lucia. *Maternity Care in a Spanish-American Community of New Mexico.* Washington, D. C., Anthropological Series, The Catholic University of America, no. 13, 1948.

[52] Watson, James B., and Julian Samora. "Subordinate Leadership in a Bicultural Community: An Analysis," *American Sociological Review,* 19 (1954): 413–421.

[53] Wyatt, Frederick. "Guidance Problems Among Student Nurses," *American Journal of Orthopsychiatry,* 17 (1947): 416–425.